Nursing &
Midwifery
UNCOVERED

Careers Uncovered guides aim to expose the truth about what it's really like to work in a particular field, containing unusual and thought-provoking facts about the profession you are interested in. Written in a lively and accessible style, *Careers Uncovered* guides explore the highs and lows of the career, along with the job opportunities and skills and qualities you will need to help you make your way forward.

Titles in this series include:

Accountancy Uncovered, 2nd edition
Art & Design Uncovered
Charity & Voluntary Work Uncovered
Design Uncovered
E-Commerce Uncovered
The Internet Uncovered
Journalism Uncovered, 2nd edition
Law Uncovered, 2nd edition
Marketing Uncovered, 2nd edition
Media Uncovered, 2nd edition
Medicine Uncovered, 2nd edition
Music Industry Uncovered, 2nd edition
Nursing & Midwifery Uncovered, 3rd edition
Performing Arts Uncovered, 2nd edition
Psychology Uncovered
Sport & Fitness Uncovered, 2nd edition
Teaching Uncovered, 2nd edition
The Travel Industry Uncovered
Working For Yourself Uncovered

Nursing & Midwifery UNCOVERED

Jim Bird & Marie Borrego

3rd edition

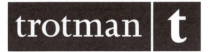
trotman | t

Nursing & Midwifery Uncovered

This third edition published in 2010 by Trotman, an imprint of Crimson Publishing, Westminster House, Kew Road, Richmond, Surrey TW9 2ND

© Trotman Publishing 2010

Authors: Jim Bird and Marie Borrego
Author of the previous edition: Laurel Alexander

First and second editions published by Trotman & Co Ltd in 2004 and 2006

© Trotman & Co Ltd 2004, 2006

British Library Cataloguing in Publication Data
A catalogue record for this book is available from the British Library

ISBN: 978-1-84455-242-9

Typeset by RefineCatch Ltd, Bungay, Suffolk

Printed and bound in the UK by Ashford Colour Press, Gosport, Hants

Contents

About the authors   vii

Acknowledgements   ix

Introduction   xi

1   What is nursing and midwifery?   1

2   Choosing your field   13

3   Adult nursing   25

4   Children's nursing   45

5   Mental health nursing   59

6   Learning disabilities nursing   75

7   Midwifery   91

8   Related career roles in nursing and midwifery   105

9   Training, skills and qualifications   113

10 How to find your first role   135

11 Career progression and future prospects   153

12 Further information   165

13 Glossary   169

About the authors

JIM BIRD

A registered nurse for more than 25 years, Jim has many years of clinical experience in a range of intensive care units and specialist cardiac and thoracic surgery units. Having worked as a staff nurse, charge nurse, education lead and service manager, for the past 15 years he has been a lecturer in nursing at the University of Southampton.

Motivated by both professionalism and the health care his family members have received, he is passionate about high-quality health care and wouldn't hesitate to recommend following a profession in health care.

MARIE BORREGO

Marie has worked as a careers adviser and team leader in Hampshire since 1987. Her work has included supporting young people in schools and colleges in Havant and Southampton. In 2005 she joined the University of Southampton where she supported a wide range of students and developed her knowledge of the health care professions through her work with student nurses, midwives, their lecturers and NHS employers. She is now Head of Careers at Peter Symonds College in Winchester.

Acknowledgements

JIM BIRD

I am very grateful for the support and patience of my wife and our four daughters in the preparation of this book and also the many students and patients who have told their personal stories. In addition, I am indebted to my parents and others who influenced my own decision to nurse and the numerous colleagues who have shaped and continue to shape my direction in and enthusiasm for professional health care.

MARIE BORREGO

Having been faced with the challenge of writing this book, I am thankful to family, friends and the health care professionals who have given me their support along the way. I would also like to thank the people who provided their case studies and particularly Clare Aspden, Supervised Practice Facilitator, Southampton University Hospitals NHS Trust and Cathy Taylor, Careers Adviser, Royal College of Nursing for their invaluable information and advice.

Introduction

Nursing and midwifery are popular careers that many consider either when they are still in full-time education or at a later stage in their lives. Sometimes even an illness or birth in a family can lead to someone deciding that they wish to join either profession. This book aims to provide you with a focused understanding of the variety of careers open to anyone wishing to train as a nurse or midwife in the UK.

The first chapter starts with definitions of the terms 'nurse', 'midwife' and a number of related job titles. A history of both professions is provided and it brings you right up to date with an understanding of the purpose of the Nursing and Midwifery Council (NMC), the professional body representing UK nurses and midwives. The chapter ends by describing how technological advances have further developed the role of today's nurses and midwives.

Where you would like to practise and the specific areas of nursing and midwifery that might suit you are important decisions that need to be made when joining either profession, and Chapter 2 deals with the many choices available.

The following five chapters focus on the role of specific nursing specialisms – adult, children's, mental health and learning disabilities – and midwifery. Each chapter highlights the duties and responsibilities undertaken by each specialist professional along with the skills they use. Real-life case studies are provided to further illustrate the breadth of responsibilities and experiences amassed by new and experienced nurses and midwives. The patient's perspective is also provided through case studies of people who have been cared for in the UK. Interwoven within each of these chapters is information about the treatment of various illnesses and explanations of the settings in which nursing and midwifery support is delivered.

In Chapter 8 we look at roles that are related to those already covered in the earlier chapters to give you an idea of the other careers you could look into if you're interested in this sector.

The general skills and initial work experience needed to train in either profession are outlined in Chapter 9. Tips are provided to help you to write an effective application for entry to a university course in nursing or midwifery. The range of educational qualifications required for entry to either profession is explained, along with the university application process and the general structure of nursing and midwifery degree courses.

Chapter 10 looks at applying for your first nursing or midwifery job. It highlights the various steps that you need to take when applying for work: how to identify your skills; CV writing; and tackling application forms. Important points such as where to look for vacancies and how to prepare for and handle interviews and assessment centres are also covered.

Career progression and future prospects in both professions are outlined in Chapter 11. The salary and career structure on offer to nurses and midwives with two or more years' experience is explained, along with information about the types of jobs available further up the career ladder.

Chapter 12 gives a number of key contacts and resources to help you plan your future career in nursing and midwifery.

Finally, we have included a glossary in Chapter 13; there might be some medical terms in this book that you haven't come across before.

Chapter One
WHAT IS NURSING AND MIDWIFERY?

Advances in training standards and increasing independence and responsibility mean that there has never been a more exciting time to become a professional nurse or midwife. The location of work is also changing, with nurses and midwives working not just in traditional hospital and community settings but also independently, in prisons, cruise ships, the armed forces and in every country in the world!

Nurse training normally takes three years, and is shared equally between university education and health care placements. Nursing has always been focused on the needs of the individual and their family rather than on specific illnesses or conditions. Nurses help people to live more comfortable and independent lives, or have a peaceful end to life, by providing physical, mental and emotional care, advice and counsel.

A midwife is normally the lead health professional supporting, guiding and caring for the pregnant mother and family until the time of birth, during the delivery itself and additionally supporting the baby and mother during the postnatal period. Midwifery training also takes three years, and is shared between university and maternal health settings, which allows the student to gain expertise in physiological assessment and the complex skills needed for physical and psychological care.

Nursing and midwifery are popular careers that many people consider either when they are still in full-time education or at a later stage in their lives. Some might have wanted to join either profession from an early age, while others will have made the decision after having worked in other occupations. Sometimes even an illness or birth in a family can lead to someone deciding that they want to become a nurse or midwife.

There are well over 600,000 professional nurses and midwives in the UK and more than 70,000 in Ireland. This means that nursing and midwifery are among the most popular careers – almost all of us can count a nurse or midwife among our relations, friends and acquaintances.

This chapter will explain what the terms 'nurse' and 'midwife' mean and help clear up some common misunderstandings. In particular, the chapter will explore how the role of nurses and midwives contributes to high-quality health care, especially the 'fit' with other health professionals and carers; and it looks at recent developments in delivering care as well as those anticipated in the future. This first chapter will also help give an overview of employment, looking both at who a future employer might be and the prospects of getting a job.

GETTING THE TERMS RIGHT

What is a nurse? What is a midwife? They sound straightforward enough, but they are widely misunderstood.

Nurse

This is called a 'protected title' – in other words it can only be used in certain circumstances. In the UK this means that the title 'nurse' can only be used by someone holding professional registration as a nurse with the regulatory body. Nurses work with people who are unwell, injured or who have health care needs due to age or disability. The care provided can be diverse, variously supporting physical, mental, psychological and/ or emotional wellbeing. Nurses work in many different settings and their roles vary enormously. Nurses train to work in one of four 'branches' of nursing: adult, child, mental health or learning disability.

Nursery nurse

Nursery nurses assist qualified staff in nurseries, schools, family centres, hospitals and private homes (as nannies), helping children under 5 years old with play, learning, social development and personal care.

Health care assistant

Health care assistants work under the supervision of other health professionals such as nurses or midwives in locations such as hospitals, community settings, nursing homes or private homes. There are many variations in the role, depending on the place of work and patient needs, but it frequently involves personal care. Some health care assistants undertake training to extend their role or to specialise – this can sometimes be a route into professional nurse training.

Carer

A carer, or young carer if under 18 years old, is someone who provides help and support to a partner, child, relation, friend or neighbour without being paid. There is more of this 'informal care' in the UK than any other type of care. Carers give assistance to people who need additional help because of age, illness or disability. This is a frequent starting point for people thinking of becoming a nurse or midwife.

Nursing (or midwifery) auxiliary

This is an older, and now less frequently used, term for a health care assistant.

Wet nurse

This is not a term used for professional care roles: it refers to a woman, often paid, who breastfeeds and cares for another's child. Wet nurses are often used in many developing countries.

Midwife

Midwives provide professional advice, care and support for women, their partners and families before, during and after the birth of their child. They support the mother in caring for the new baby during its first 28 days of life. Midwives are personally responsible for the health of both mother and child, working in multi-professional teams in hospital and, in recent years, increasingly in a variety of community health care settings. The title 'midwife' is a protected title.

Health visitor

Health visitors are qualified nurses or midwives who have completed further specialist training. The role of a health visitor is to work as a lead member of the primary health care team, and they are concerned with promoting optimal health and preventing ill health. While they work with all age groups, in reality most of the work is targeted at supporting families and young children from shortly after birth. Health visitors work extensively with other professionals from backgrounds such as health (including nurses and midwives), education, welfare, housing and other social support services.

THE START OF NURSING AND MIDWIFERY

It is often helpful to understand the background of a subject in order to help place it in the contemporary context.

When people think of the history of nursing, they often recall the outstanding contributions made by such well-known figures as Florence Nightingale ('the lady with the lamp') and Mary Seacole. However, present-day nursing and midwifery has much earlier roots. One of the first recorded mentions of nursing dates from 250 BC, when what is believed to be the world's first nursing school started in India. It appears that only men were considered 'pure' enough to become nurses. Early Sanskrit writings highlighted the personal characteristics necessary for a nurse, such as kindness, together with essential patient skills such as cleverness and skills in every service a patient might require, including competency in cooking, bathing and washing the patient, rubbing and massaging limbs, lifting and assisting patients to walk, making and cleaning beds … and more! A well-known story in the New Testament describes the 'good Samaritan', who recovered an injured traveller and then paid an innkeeper to provide further care for the injured man; again it seems that a man was paid to provide nursing care.

Towards the end of the Roman Empire, plagues afflicted much of Europe and an estimated 10% of the population died. At this time a number of groups, often men, were established to provide care and nursing to those affected. These included the Parabolani (AD 300) and the Benedictine nursing order. Throughout the Middle Ages it is recorded that mainly men provided nursing care: nursing organisations included the Knights Hospitallers (distant forerunners of today's St John Ambulance Brigade); and St Camillus initiated the use of the red cross symbol and the first ambulance service.

There is little evidence that the roles of nursing or organised caring kept up with the advances of medicine through the centuries, perhaps in part because such care was often undertaken by the military or by religious orders – both of which required a lifetime commitment. The poor state of affairs in nursing in Europe in the 18th century is apparent from records of those providing nursing care being illiterate and of governments staffing hospitals by recruiting thieves, prostitutes and drunks to provide nursing as an alternative to serving jail sentences! Not surprisingly, this resulted in nursing services being highly unsatisfactory, poorly organised and unreliable. Death rates were appalling and infection was common in what today would be uninhabitable ward areas that were covered in filth, lacking sanitation or clean water and infested with insects and lice.

The development of modern nursing can be traced to the 19th century with the renewal of some religious orders such as the Sisters of Charity and the foundation of civilian orders such as the Red Cross, established in Switzerland in 1863.

The best known nurse in history is undoubtedly Florence Nightingale, a well-educated Englishwoman who was born into a family of high social standing. The reforms of Florence Nightingale are well worth reviewing briefly as they form the basis for today's contemporary nursing practice.

Florence Nightingale was born in 1820. She wanted to be a nurse but was discouraged by her parents, as nursing was then perceived to be a job for people of low class who were not worthy of more reputable work. After visiting Kaiserswerth, an institute in Germany, Florence Nightingale was inspired by the way in which care was organised there. She was so challenged by the limited training provided for the nurses (deaconesses) that she toured other European hospital establishments to learn how the preparation and teaching of nurses might be improved. On returning to England in 1853 she had the opportunity to put into practice some of the concepts she had learned when she supervised the Establishment for Gentlewomen during Illness, a nursing home in London for women of limited resources. It was here that the early Nightingale principles of cleanliness, fresh air, hygiene and what we would now call 'holistic care' were demonstrated and proven to benefit patients.

In 1854, following public outcry at the lack of health care for soldiers following major battles, the British government asked Florence

Nightingale to take over organising and directing the nursing care of sick and injured soldiers in the Crimean War. She went, with almost 40 nurses, to Scutari, a Russian city, where she found the hospitals in a very poor state – dirty ward areas, infestations (beds, patients and staff) of lice and insects, inadequate catering and diet, dire sanitation and an almost total absence of laundry facilities for bedding and clothing. She worked hard, often at odds with the military and governmental establishment, to improve conditions in the hospitals. The improvements she initiated, especially in sanitation, training, clinical and psychosocial care, led to hospital mortality dropping from over 40% to around 2%. Not surprisingly, she became very popular with the British public.

Returning to England after the Crimean War, Florence Nightingale was extensively involved in reorganising hospital services and establishing the formal training of nurses, based on her 1859 publication, *Notes on Nursing: What it is and what it is not.* She defined nursing as an art which, 'like any other art requires a sense of calling and diligent apprenticeship'; for many years this was the foundation of nurse training all over the world. For at least the next hundred years the key principles of Florence Nightingale's first nursing school were widely replicated. These principles included: '(1) nurses should be technically and theoretically trained in hospitals, which are equipped for this purpose and (2) nurses should live in homes so designed as to promote good moral life and discipline'. Her principles are still the ethical basis for the nursing profession.

The history of midwifery is also ancient: it goes back at least to ancient Greece, whose laws required that midwives must have had children themselves. The attitudes of society towards midwives have varied throughout history: in 16th-century Europe, childbirth was viewed as one of the 'diseases of women'. The first school for midwives was established in Paris in the early 16th century. Jane Sharp, an English midwife, wrote in 1671 of some sound key principles, such as not hurrying labour; but, in a rather restrictive tone, she also warned midwives against theoretical knowledge. Later, in the 18th century, midwives were advised (1724) to have the qualities of being 'grave, considerate, patient, meek and not too fat'. However, the skills of midwives were recognised in 1735 by Edmund Chapman, a strong advocate for midwifery and an early user of obstetric forceps, who described midwifery as 'one of the most noble …

operations. [It] requires judgment for there is generally one and often two lives snatched from the jaws of death.'

Midwifery has, like nursing, developed from male-dominated medical systems to the modern, often female-led, community that helps women throughout pregnancy and childbirth. Childbirth in the 19th century was marked by a contrast between the middle and upper classes, who preferred expensive, doctor-led obstetric care, and the working classes, who had no choice but to make use of traditional care from midwives. Towards the end of the 19th century nurses began to be trained as midwives (1862), and the Midwives Institute was established in 1881. The 1902 Midwives Act established midwifery as a profession in Great Britain, with training supervised and registration formally recorded. Despite clinical advances, for example the use of equipment such as forceps, and the development of the profession, pregnant women continued to receive very little care before labour itself had commenced.

NURSING AND MIDWIFERY TODAY

While there is value in learning how nursing and midwifery have developed, of course current practice has changed and developed dramatically in the last 20 or 30 years. That is not to say that everything has changed. Patients nowadays often have the same problems as patients of 100 years ago – pain, discomfort, loss of independence – and nurses and midwives continue to need many of the same characteristics and skills – caring, listening, nurturing and much more.

However, the way in which nurses and midwives work has changed radically, as have their responsibilities, job titles, employers and accountability. Much of this change has come about with the increased professionalisation of nursing and midwifery, technical advances in health care, improved training and changes in public expectations, including cost-effectiveness.

Professionalism

In the not too distant past nurses and midwives were frequently portrayed in the media, in film and television dramas as 'angels' who could do no wrong; or as people of 'low virtue' in slapstick-style comedy. Of course, neither extreme was ever accurate, but one thing that is clear is that nursing and midwifery have changed from being a role or vocation to being a profession.

Defining a profession or professionalism is not always straightforward: the words have meant different things at different times; and nurses and midwives themselves, together with the society in which they work, have modified their ideas as society itself has changed.

Formal registration and recognition is far from new. The UK register of midwives was established in 1902 and nurse registration in 1919. In 1983 the UK's Central Council for Nursing, Midwifery and Health Visiting was established to maintain a formal register of UK nurses, midwives and health visitors; provide guidance to those on the registers; and investigate and manage complaints about registrants. Also in 1983 a national board was established for each of the four UK countries; their key functions were to monitor the quality of nursing and midwifery education courses. In 2002, the functions of the UKCC and many national board responsibilities were taken over by a new Nursing and Midwifery Council (NMC); a number of substantial reforms to training (Project 2000) were embedded in practice.

The primary purpose of the NMC is to safeguard the health and wellbeing of the public. The key functions include the following:

- registration of all nurses and midwives in the UK to ensure they are properly qualified and competent to work

- setting the standards of education, training and conduct that nurses and midwives need to deliver high-quality health care consistently throughout their careers

- ensuring that nurses and midwives keep their skills and knowledge up to date and uphold the standards of their professional code; this is achieved by annual re-registration processes

- ensuring that midwives are safe to practise by setting rules for their practice and supervision

- using fair processes to investigate allegations made against nurses and midwives who may not have followed the code of professional standards.

Some of the key professional attributes that nurses and midwives must possess are accountability, knowledge and autonomy.

Accountability

This refers to the practitioner's 'answerability' for their own actions – in other words, accepting the consequences of one's behaviour. For both nurses and midwives, accountability for practice includes knowing your limitations: not doing more than your experience or training allows; providing input into decisions that affect practice (such as staffing levels); advancing standards of care and setting quality standards; being responsible with personal information, for example confidential personal records.

Knowledge

The basis of professional practice, knowledge enables nurses and midwives to define the nature of problems, identify solutions, make autonomous (individual) decisions and use intuition in their practice. The 'body of knowledge' to enhance care includes:

- theory, practice and clinical knowledge

- the ability to apply knowledge to a variety of situations

- asking questions to expand and extend knowledge

- efficiently and effectively acquiring information

- using evidence from other disciplines or professional groups

- sharing/communicating knowledge with colleagues and patients/families.

Autonomy

This means working independently. The nurse or midwife makes decisions within their scope of practice, i.e. within the limits of their experience, training and 'up to datedness'. It includes the capacity of the nurse or midwife to determine their own course of action and make their own decisions. Many midwives have worked autonomously for many years and in recent years this has become much more common for nurses.

Technical advances

The pace of technical change in professional health care is a fast one! For example, improved medications and treatments have led to survival rates for some types of childhood leukaemia rising to up to 90% in the UK; survival from major trauma and serious illness is hugely improved with the use of highly sophisticated and often invasive monitoring and life support systems. In surgery, advances in instrumentation and anaesthesia mean that procedures once thought of only in science fiction are now routinely carried out, for example repairs to the heart without opening the chest and neurosurgery on people who are awake.

Such technological advances inevitably have many consequences for nurses. One key effect is that hospitals are now considered to be places for the very unwell and those having more complex treatment or investigation. Advances in treatment mean that more people survive illnesses that would have limited their life expectancy only a few years ago. A good example of this is management of the common lung disorder chronic obstructive pulmonary disease (COPD), often linked to smoking. Advances in managing COPD, especially with more effective use of medications and very short hospital admissions for acute exacerbations such as pneumonia, have led to many people with COPD living much longer and being able to live at home for longer. This means that there are now many more people living in the community with health conditions that, although serious, are not immediately life threatening; on the other hand, the conditions don't go away and need continuing care. Such conditions are often called 'long-term conditions', and this is a significant area for future nursing practice in the community. It is likely that in the future there will be a modest number of hospitals for the most ill patients, and that a much larger number of people with long-term conditions will be routinely managed by nurses, and through minor exacerbations of their illness, in the community. Long-term conditions, for people of all ages, often managed by nurses in the community include:

- lung conditions such as COPD and asthma

- metabolic disorders such as diabetes

- vascular problems such as poor circulation to the feet, leg ulcers

- heart failure

■   epilepsy, multiple sclerosis and other neurological conditions

■   many mental health conditions

■   cancer

■   joint disorders such as osteo-arthritis and rheumatoid arthritis

■   disability from acute illnesses such as stroke.

To summarise, nursing and midwifery have certainly come a long way! Even in the 30 years this author has been a nurse, the changes have been both dramatic and very welcome. Nursing and midwifery have been transformed from traditional, institutionalised careers to dynamic, forward-thinking professions with an extensive evidence base for delivering care, and considerable autonomy and independence in clinical practice. Of course, change has not stopped: over the next few years there will be further advances in both education and practice; and as health care systems are reformed to improve efficiency, there will be greater opportunities for nurses and midwives to be at the very forefront of delivering care.

Chapter Two
CHOOSING YOUR FIELD

If you want to go into either nursing or midwifery, you will be faced with a number of opportunities to choose from. In either professional group, your initial choice of field of practice and training will allow you to make choices in the future, including:

- employer

- specific area of work

- community or hospital setting

- specialised training

- opportunities for travel

- higher academic study or research.

Unlike many professions, in nursing in particular there are frequently opportunities to make new choices throughout your career. Marlyn's story on the next page is an example.

EMPLOYERS

For many years, public perception has often regarded the traditional employer of nurses and midwives as the National Health Service (NHS) in the UK or the Health Services Executive (HSE) in Ireland. While this

Marlyn, aged 28, is a mental health nurse.

case STUDY

Having qualified in 2003, I worked for five years in a psychiatric admissions unit, supporting clients of all ages through their acute episodes of illness. One of my key roles was in establishing patient-centred care and accurate observation and assessment of patients who were sometimes very low in mood, and not interested in my intention to support them back to good health. Patients often had major diagnoses of illnesses such as schizophrenia, bipolar disorder, compulsive behaviour and substance misuse, and had sometimes tried to harm themselves. As my experience increased I began to identify that for a number of patients their illness was associated with the grief of bereavement. Pursuing this growing interest, I furthered my studies with degree-level specialist studies in loss, combining this with bereavement counselling qualifications. I now work for a charity as a nurse specialist in bereavement counselling. Mostly working independently, I support people in the community where loss is associated with mental ill health, helping to prevent acute exacerbations or hospital admissions and to maintain independent living.

is certainly a big part of the employment picture it is certainly not the whole picture.

Who employs nurses and midwives?

NHS	Nurses	410,000
	Midwives	19,000
Armed forces (UK)	Nurses	2,800 (estimate)
Independent health providers	Nurses	80,000 (estimate)
HSE (Ireland)	Nurses	60,000

Other major employers include charities, local authorities or councils, the prison service and police, industry/commerce, nursing homes, and education and research providers such as universities.

SOME INITIAL QUESTIONS

If you are thinking about a career in nursing or midwifery it is worth asking yourself some questions well before you consider applying for a place at university. The following might be helpful as prompts, but don't feel compelled to go through them rigidly – the idea is to help you think about your options as early as you can.

I know that I enjoy caring, but how can I be sure about full-blown nursing?
Many people enjoy caring, they feel it is part of their nature or who they are – some call it their 'vocation'. There are many jobs and professions that involve caring, for example all health professions, teaching, police, animal care, gardening, social work … and many more.

People can change from one profession/career to another, but it can be difficult. It is worth listening to what your close friends/family/work colleagues think – what sort of person do they see you as? This is where work experience (through school/college or what you arrange yourself), voluntary work or perhaps temporary employment can be really useful in helping you distinguish between perhaps two possible choices.

There are lots of different health professions: how can I choose between them?
In addition to the four areas of nursing and midwifery there are many other health professions. These include some which are significantly clinical or 'hands on' – e.g. occupational therapy, medicine, physiotherapy, podiatry, psychotherapy, radiography, paramedic work, dietetics/nutrition, speech and language therapy, dental surgery, psychology – and others which involve less face-to-face contact with patients, e.g. pharmacy, pathology, lab technology.

Read carefully about the professional groups you are interested in – narrow the field. In particular, look at what people in the job actually do. Does it interest you? Does it match your ambitions? Does it match your own set of skills? To help make a final choice, experience is really helpful, whether it's work shadowing, voluntary work or paid work. In addition, you might be able to observe friends or family receiving care, for example through hospital visiting or, with their permission, accompany them to treatments/tests.

Is nursing/midwifery too academic for me?

In order to train successfully, and then register as a nurse or midwife (in the UK and Ireland) students must pass both the academic and clinical (placement) halves of their course. This is very important to universities as it in their interests to take on successful students who have the academic capability to study to bachelor's or first-degree level.

Ask your teacher/tutor for their predictions for your current or future pre-university courses, matching this against your own realistic ambitions. You can then explore the entry grades for universities (e.g. via UCAS). There can be considerable variation; for example, at the time of writing GCE A level (or equivalent) entry grades for an adult nursing degree at UK universities ranged from two subjects each at grade D to three subjects each at grade B. It is also well worth visiting a university open day to talk to tutors. If you don't think you are adequately prepared for a course you can either plan to upgrade your qualifications or enter nursing/midwifery care through employment and training as a health care assistant.

Is my maths good enough?

For all nurses and midwives, accuracy in dispensing medications and calculating or checking dosages is an absolute essential. A misplaced decimal point could mean a patient gets 10 times too much or 10 times too little medication – either could have very serious consequences. The NMC sets minimum standards for number skills which universities apply to their applicants. The issue is more than having an exam pass – it is about being comfortable with handling numbers. In reality, the arithmetic is very straightforward – simple addition, subtraction, multiplication and division – it just needs to be done with a high degree of accuracy.

The entry standard is currently set at minimum grade C in GCSE Mathematics; a grade D is not accepted. Alternative number-related qualifications are considered by some universities – check on an individual basis.

All university nursing and midwifery courses include content that is specific to calculating drug dosages – before you start your course you are expected to be competent with numbers. Many universities now ask applicants to sit a short number or maths assessment as part of their selection day activities.

Is my English good enough?

Accurate oral and written communication skills are essential in nursing and midwifery. The NMC has minimum standards for competence in the English language, which universities follow. Universities in the UK and Ireland teach and examine primarily in English; each institution will want to be confident of your competence. In addition, universities in Wales and Ireland may prefer or require students to have competence in Welsh or Irish.

The entry standard is currently assessed at GCSE English Language, grade C or better; a grade D is not accepted. A number of alternative English language qualifications are considered by some universities – check on an individual basis.

If English is not your first language – for example if the main language of your home country or education was not English – different requirements apply. Check with universities and/or the NMC website.

Many universities now ask applicants to sit a short written assessment as part of selection day activities.

How common is it for men to become nurses and midwives?

All areas of nursing and midwifery are open to and are practised by both men and women. Between 5% and 10% of all nurses are male (UK/Ireland); there are very few male midwives.

Men and women have equal opportunity to train and register as a nurse or midwife. Historically, a slightly higher proportion of men work in mental health nursing.

How on earth do I decide between adult, child, mental health and learning disability nursing?

Most, but not quite all, universities, require you to apply for a specific area of nursing in your initial application. This is because the health service works with universities to forward plan its workforce needs – i.e.

it calculates and plans for specific numbers of nurses to qualify three or four years ahead.

You will probably need to consider several points.

1   Your initial motivation to nurse: some people have a specific 'trigger' experience.

2   Your own personality. How do you 'get on' with different age groups/ different people's needs?

3   Experience: if at all possible, gain shadowing/work/voluntary/ employed experience in more than one setting if you are not certain.

Can I change between different areas of nursing?

Within the university training period this can be difficult and is certainly not guaranteed – in fact it can be impossible.

There are a few, very limited opportunities to gain an additional registration after qualifying. This might lead to a nurse being dual qualified, for example holding both adult and mental health registrations, or adult nursing and midwifery. You should not rely on dual registration being available – the funding and availability of the relevant courses can and does change, largely depending on workforce planning and economic factors.

Prepare carefully to be sure of your preferred area of practice before you apply. Experience (see above) is frequently the deciding factor.

I really enjoy working with young children. Is midwifery or child nursing more relevant?

Chapters 4 and 7 of this book should be helpful. Midwives' primary role is supporting women through pregnancy and birth and helping the new mums to look after their own children – there is little direct child care involved. Children's nurses work with unwell children of all ages, who often behave very differently from healthy children; it is important to remember that most of their time is spent with children who are ill, very ill or disabled by their health.

If you want to work with healthy, well children you could consider a role in teaching, nursery care or play. If necessary, work experience (see above) will allow you to explore the nature of child nursing and midwifery practices.

I seem to get on well with older adults, at least socially. Which area of nursing will suit me best?

Chapters 3 and 5 of this book should help. In both adult and mental health nursing, many of the patients or clients are older – 70, 80 years or more. While both types of nursing support people with their physical and mental health needs, adult nurses specialise in supporting physiological needs and mental health nurses are specially skilled in the care of psychological need, including dementia.

Gaining experience (see above) is likely to be very useful; consider getting some insight into or familiarity with a community hospital or nursing home, both of which will often care for older adults with physical and mental health needs.

Do I need a nursing registration to support people who have a learning disability?

The short answer is yes and no! Learning disability nurses specialise in supporting people with a learning disability, with a particular focus on health needs. Other professional groups support the same clients, and those with fewer health needs. Examples include social workers, speech and language therapists and housing advisers.

Gaining experience (see above) is likely to be very useful; consider getting some insight into a community unit or through activities of charities that support clients. You might also want to consider mental health nursing, in which your skills in supporting clients with challenging behaviours will be developed.

Should I choose a diploma or a degree?

In Scotland, Wales and Ireland the only preparation available for nurse or midwife registration is at first degree level. In England, midwifery training is at degree level only. All English nurse training is currently planned to follow suit by 2013, and many universities will be 'degree only' before this.

Your choice of course must be the right one for you. Because the level of academic assessment is slightly lower for Diploma and Advanced Diploma courses, entry grades tend to be a little lower: so while this entry route remains available it is a good option for some people.

In the long term, nursing is moving to become an all-graduate profession, reflecting the complexity of care, need for accountability

and decision making and increasing dependency of patients.
For nurses who register with diploma-level preparation there are
many opportunities to 'top up' to a degree – this is taken up by an
increasingly large number of nurses.

Can I become a nurse through the armed forces?

The UK armed forces support a small number of undergraduate
nurses each year, and these places are always oversubscribed. Student
places for adult and mental health nursing are available; all students
are salaried for the duration of their course. Initial basic military training
precedes nurse training alongside other nursing students at a single
university.

For students with aspirations to work as a nurse in the armed forces,
this is a great opportunity and financially more secure than other
options. However, only certain people will find it appealing, and the
selection process is rigorous. More detailed information is available
though the armed forces websites.

What is best: a three- or four-year course?

The majority of UK universities offer both nursing and midwifery on
three-year courses, with some opportunities for nursing over four
years. As course content will be the same, course length is a personal
choice – the four-year variant has longer vacations with perhaps more
opportunity for paid holiday employment, but it obviously takes a year
longer before registration.

It is worth exploring the opportunities available at your preferred
universities and discussing any financial implications with your family.

Professionally, the length of course is neither an advantage nor a
disadvantage.

I think I might want to teach nursing/midwifery in the future. Does my choice of course matter?

Nurses and midwives are employed as lecturers in universities (to
teach and as researchers); and in colleges (sixth form and further
education), especially supporting health and social care programmes.
University lecturers normally have a higher degree at master's or
doctoral level; college lecturers will be graduates. In either setting an
additional teaching qualification is often necessary.

All fields of practice – in both nursing and midwifery – can lead to employment as a lecturer. It is likely that you will need at least several years of experience working in your field before full-time teaching becomes possible. All areas of practice/employment can be useful preparation for subsequent work as a lecturer.

If I want to work in industry as an occupational health nurse, how should I prepare?

Occupational health nurses work in many sectors, including traditional heavy industry (trauma, health and safety, health screening, first aid and training) and also state and commercial employers (health screening, fitness to work or disability assessment). Most occupational health nurses are adult trained, though a few have a background in mental health nursing; additional specialist training is available.

This is not a straightforward area in which to gain experience but it is worth contacting large employers in your area. The Royal College of Nursing (RCN) has a useful specialist interest group.

Am I too old (or too young) to start nursing or midwifery?

The simple answer, for the UK at least, is 'no'! The UK regulator, the NMC, complies with age discrimination legislation by not setting an age limit on entry to training; all UK universities apply this. That said, it is normal practice for new entrants to complete at least sixth-form study before starting their training. While many students are aged between 18 and 20 when they start, many others commence after a career break or to change professional direction; such students may well be in their 30s, 40s or older when they start.

Age is not a factor in starting nurse or midwifery training, but you do need to be physically mature and fit (an occupational health assessment is undertaken) and give the university confidence that you can complete the course. For young people, it is often useful to spend time gaining experience before starting a course. For others, especially if they have not done any formal study for some years, updating their learning skills might be needed, for example completing an Access to Higher Education course or distance learning programme (e.g. with the Open University).

Do I have to be good at science?

All nursing courses involve strong elements of physiology or life science; and there is increased emphasis on anatomy and physiology in midwifery.

You will need a science to at least GCSE grade C or better. Some universities may require a higher grade or preparation at a higher level (e.g. GCE A level).

Before committing to any further science study it is well worth seeking advice from your preferred universities – some institutions advise avoiding certain programmes. In the main, where additional preparation is needed, courses which are widely considered to be suitable include human biology/physiology, some distance learning programmes (e.g. the Open University) and science-based Access to Higher Education courses.

Do I need to do further training after I have registered?
All nurses and midwives need to keep up to date with current best practice based on best available evidence; annual updating is compulsory. Many registered nurses and midwives become mentors, supporting and assessing students in training. In addition, many nurses and midwives undertake further training in their specialist field, either through short courses or through longer courses with recordable qualifications. Many courses are undertaken in collaboration between the employer and local university.

Most nurses and midwives undertake additional training to extend their skills and knowledge – this is a career-long approach.

EXPERIENCE

When you are making a choice about which field of health care to seek your career in, the value of experience is worth emphasising because it:

- helps you observe or engage in the reality of practice

- lets you engage with 'real' current practitioners

- introduces you to the patient/client group(s)

- helps you experience the highs and lows of health care

- is often a key trigger in your decision making.

Opportunities for experience

■ Many college and sixth-form students have the opportunity of work experience placements; where possible these should be carefully chosen to support your potential interest, even if you have to arrange them yourself.

■ Voluntary work: perhaps after school/college or during vacation periods. Ideally, you should sustain volunteering for a period of time (months or more), taking care that it doesn't interfere with any studies.

■ Employment: for example part-time work in a local nursing home or Sure Start centre; alternatively, on a casual basis with local employers or care agencies.

■ Potential adult nurse? Consider: nursing home; residential home; day centre; community hospital; general hospital; support charities; community care groups; homeless shelter; family members.

■ Potential children's nurse? Consider: special school; support groups for disabled children; nursery or holiday play schemes for children with physical, behavioural or other needs.

■ Potential mental health nurse? Consider: nursing home; residential home; day centre; community hospital; support charities; community care group; homeless shelter; family members.

■ Potential learning disability nurse? Consider: residential settings; day centre; supported employment settings; supported learning facilities; support charities; community care groups; homeless shelter; family members.

■ Potential midwife? Consider: talking to a midwife you are acquainted with; assisting at local antenatal classes; observing or engaging with pre-natal support offered by self-help or charitable groups; accompanying a friend or relation to their pre- and/or postnatal appointments.

For more details on gaining work experience turn to page 114.

FURTHER INFORMATION

You may well want to pursue your thinking about choices further. Useful sources of information include the following.

- University open days (if higher education is needed for professional preparation): check individual universities' websites. Current students and staff are often available, and talks and demonstrations may be on offer.

- Hospital and care provider open days: most large health care employers offer at least an annual open day where departmental staff are available to demonstrate and explain their roles. See local newspapers/radio or enquire at the hospital's press or media office.

- Current practitioners: it is likely that you or someone in your family already knows several nurses or midwives. These are useful people to build a friendship with and to ask questions that you might find awkward or embarrassing in front of a larger audience.

Chapter Three
ADULT NURSING

WHAT DO ADULT NURSES DO?

Adult nurses deliver specialist nursing to people aged over 18 (or 16). Sometimes considered to be 'general nursing', adult nursing is certainly broad, but in reality it goes well beyond anything that might be considered 'general', as adult nurses have a diverse range of specialist professional skills.

The care that adult nurses give includes:

- assessing patient need, using a proven research-based tool or protocol
- monitoring clinical information, e.g. blood pressure, blood oxygen saturations
- physical examinations such as auscultation, venous return
- prescribing medication
- administering drugs, injections, nutritional supplements
- using evidence-based practice to assess, plan and deliver care of wounds and ulcers
- administering blood transfusions and intravenous fluids
- basic or advanced resuscitation
- using complex life support equipment
- helping patients meet their personal needs, such as washing and toileting

- participating in or leading patient case reviews

- decision making

- engaging confidently in the network of communication around each patient

- extended skills, e.g. intubation, cannulation/venesection, taking and interpreting ECGs

- planning discharge or transfers from institutions

- palliative care

- mentoring junior staff and students

- teaching/educating patients, families and others.

Adult nurses provide care to support patients suffering from critical and urgent illness, long-term conditions, illnesses and diseases, and those requiring surgery. As with other fields of nursing care, a key focus is to provide a holistic and evidence-based programme of professional nursing care. They aim to focus on the needs of the patient rather than the illness or condition and also have key roles in promoting good health and wellbeing through education. As with other areas of nursing practice, adult nurses plan and deliver care within a multidisciplinary or interprofessional team; they are frequently the main point of contact with patients. Although working in a team is common practice, a number of adult nurses work independently within those teams, for example community matrons and a range of specialist practitioners.

Ill health: the figures

Many people face physical ill health at some point during their lifetime. Here are some figures relating to ill health in the UK.

- Over 17 million people have at least one long-term condition.

- About 2% of the population suffer from visible psoriasis.

- Approximately 300,000 people each year are diagnosed with cancer.

- The NHS has over 160,000 hospital patient beds.

- 60% of hospital beds are occupied by people with a long-term condition.

- About 30,000 serious personal injuries occur at work each year, in addition to approximately 120,000 less serious but treatable injuries.

- Chronic illness accounts for 85% of UK deaths.

- There are approximately 170,000 beds in registered nursing homes.

- Premature deaths from cardiovascular disease costs the UK around £2 billion each year.

- Each year around 40,000 people get appendicitis.

- Around two-thirds of the whole UK health budget goes to treat or care for people with long-term conditions.

James is a senior charge nurse in a hospital respiratory unit.

case STUDY

Now 40, I have worked in a number of acute and critical care environments in general hospitals, yet in my book, my career in caring started many years before. When I was a teenager, I helped my mum care for my grandparents – her parents – as they were both in their 80s and increasingly reliant on other people. Whilst my mother visited twice a day to clean, help them get up in the morning, prepare meals, etc., my role was to go into their home each day after school to get their sandwiches out of the fridge, make a cup of tea, stoke the fire and read the paper to them. While not quite as exciting as the things some of my friends did (although I wasn't exactly first pick for any sports team), I really enjoyed helping my grandparents; I like to think that I gave something to them, something that made a real difference to them.

My grandfather was often talking about his time volunteering for a national uniformed first aid organisation and I started this too. I guess it was for two reasons: one, I liked the first aid and was quite good at it; and two, I got into football matches, speedway and stock car racing – free!

After short-term jobs in a laboratory and working as a milkman I started my nurse training. Back then it wasn't adult nursing but 'general nursing', yet I spent almost all my time with adult patients. After I qualified I found my first post in an intensive care unit on nights; my friends said it was too specialist for a first nursing job, but I learned a tremendous amount here, as not only did I learn many complex technical skills but I also discovered innumerable links between my class-learned physiology and the signs, symptoms and observations of the patient before me – this I found very exciting!

After three years in two different intensive care units, I undertook a specialist respiratory course and for the last 15 years have worked in hospital respiratory units, supporting patients with severe illness such as emphysema, asthma, chest trauma including stabbing, lung cancer and pneumonia. Now a senior charge nurse, I hope in future to broaden my skills further and work as a respiratory nurse specialist in the community.

A fundamental point to consider when thinking about becoming an adult nurse is that the people they support are usually unwell. Some areas of nursing or health care focus on psychological or social aspects of health – these are very important – but for adult nurses, much time is spent supporting people who are physically ill.

We all come across people with physical health needs, probably most days. We know this because in many western countries, including the UK and Ireland, people seem to enjoy talking about health – either their own or that of people they know. Most of us will have had conversations with friends, family or work colleagues in which the topic comes around to being off school or work; an accident, a serious illness, cancer and so on. Of course, adult nurses work well beyond such conversations – one of their fundamental roles is to be 'hands on' with their patients, literally using their hands to care by undertaking personal care, assessments, administering treatments, using monitoring and life support equipment and much more.

As in all areas of nursing, if you study to become an adult nurse your curriculum will include physiology and life sciences; social sciences such as psychology, sociology and behavioural science; communication; pharmacology; and health services.

Leonard, aged 58, heart attack patient.

At 57 years old, I was beginning to make plans for an early retirement from a lifetime working as an accountant. Fit and healthy, if a little overweight, I had stopped smoking on my 40th birthday and enjoyed good food and the occasional drink. I considered myself to be in the prime of life, a successful professional – being an accountant is not seen as 'sexy' by some people, but I enjoyed the cut and thrust of deadlines, organising very large budgets and getting things right.

I particularly enjoyed the department's Christmas meal; each year we saved from summer onwards to have an outstanding spread at a classy hotel, most of us staying the night to avoid driving after a drink. Last year, as with all others, the meal was great, although returning to our room very late, I felt I had indigestion, bad enough to make me take the lift rather than use the stairs.

In the morning I still had the indigestion, it hurt – bad – and that was just in bed. Thinking it might be helpful to use the lavatory I swung myself out of bed, stood up holding my stomach, then felt a tremendous and indescribable pain; this wasn't just my stomach, now it was my chest, it felt like someone was squeezing me so tight that there wasn't any room left in my chest – it was burning me, crushing me and making me feel very black – I couldn't see anything. It must only have been there for half a minute or so – I can't remember more because the next I knew I was in hospital.

In the coronary care unit (CCU) the nurse told me I had had a heart attack, a myocardial infarction, and had only managed to get to hospital because the hotel had an automated defibrillator; the staff and paramedics had managed to restart my heart after a cardiac arrest. No wonder I couldn't remember. I was in coronary care for 10 days and began to feel a lot better, although my angiogram test showed that my coronary arteries weren't too good. When I first arrived I was given an angioplasty to reopen a coronary artery that was almost completely blocked – the one that gave me the heart attack; however, the other two main arteries supplying my heart were also bad, and angioplasty wasn't suitable. I am now waiting for an urgent triple bypass operation which should correct my heart plumbing problem.

I have been very impressed with the staff team I have seen in CCU – nurses, doctors, physiological technicians, dietitian, health care assistants, pharmacist, radiographers – then there are all the theatre, A&E and paramedic teams. When I get fully fit again I hope to do some fundraising for the CCU or one of the heart charities – they have been really good to me!

Adult nurses supported Leonard:

■ by resuscitation (including CPR) in the emergency department, administering essential drugs, setting up and reading an ECG, maintaining airway and intubation, keeping records, contacting his wife, taking blood to assess oxygen saturation, working with cardiac arrest team, transferring him safely to the CCU

■ in the CCU: continually monitoring ECG, frequently assessing blood pressure and respiration, providing personal care until independent, making a detailed admission assessment, reassuring him about his future lifestyle, providing heart education (including preparation for procedures), administering intravenous fluids/drugs and other medication, collaborating with multidisciplinary team, liaising with his wife and, by having shared discussion about activity levels, preparing him for discharge home.

ADULT NURSES WITHIN THE HEALTH CARE SYSTEM

Until recently, most people in developed countries associated being physically unwell with a formal and structured doctor-led health service; if we became unwell we saw a doctor who either treated us or arranged for us to be treated in hospital. In the UK, the established system for organising health care is as follows.

■ **Primary health care** is the first point of consultation; typically a GP/ family doctor, dentist, ophthalmic service or pharmacist. About 90% of all NHS patient contacts occur in primary care.

■ **Secondary health care** includes services that are routinely provided by general hospitals following referral by a primary care practitioner. For 'adult' care this includes management of many long-term conditions such as arthritis or heart failure, investigation and non-specialist surgery.

■ **Tertiary services** are provided by specialist, often regional, hospitals equipped with diagnostic and treatment facilities not available at local hospitals. These typically include services such as neurosurgery and renal dialysis.

Whilst this model of care has been and continues to be very successful, there are important factors that are driving changes relevant to adult nursing.

- Hospital care is very expensive: it costs around £600 per day just to stay in a hospital bed, and the cost of treatment, surgery, tests and medication need to be added to this.

- Treatments are increasingly successful: people are now much more likely to survive serious illness or trauma. This, with the general rise in life expectancy, means that the health needs of the ageing population are escalating and will continue to do so.

- Hospitals are for people who are ill or very ill, people who are not always able to fight infections. Where possible, avoiding hospital helps decrease further acquisition of infection.

- For many people, especially the old and frail, being in hospital disrupts routine. Unfamiliar surroundings often increase confusion, and distance from home means that family or friends cannot easily offer personal support.

Because of these and many other factors, there is now a steady shift in the emphasis of care towards the community, with people who would previously have been occupying a general hospital bed now being cared for in their own homes. Many of these people have at least one long-term condition, or health disruptions which are often lifelong and limit the quality of life; such conditions mostly cannot be cured but can be controlled. Many long-term conditions are regarded as a 'hidden disability'. However, those affected often experience severe limitations on their lifestyles – they have difficulty with personal care, mobility and daily activities, such as getting dressed, housework or preparing a meal.

A key adult nursing role, for example that of a community matron, is to support patients remaining in their own home rather than being admitted to hospital; this is achieved by assessing need, planning care, providing support and facilitating care by other agencies, and delivering complex and often specialist care, for example intravenous infusions/drugs and respiratory support equipment.

CONDITIONS TREATED BY ADULT NURSES

As can be seen from the paragraphs below, long-term conditions are not necessarily associated with ageing but do occur more often, and last longer, in an ageing population.

Circulation problems

In total, if hypertension (high blood pressure) is included, about 25% of the UK population have a circulatory problem. While some can be sudden and fatal, the majority can be controlled long term. Specific examples include stroke (2% of the population), heart failure, angina (5%) and having an abnormal heart rhythm (5%). In the community, as well as managing and directing treatment, adult nurses can help influence the associated physical and lifestyle risk factors such as blood lipid (fat) levels, smoking, raised blood pressure, diabetes, obesity and physical activity. The risk of these diseases increases with age, with women generally at lower risk than men until after the menopause. Nurse-led assessment – in the person's home or at a clinic – may include periodic monitoring of blood pressure, body mass (weight), blood tests (for lipids) and lifestyle/dietary/smoking evaluation; this adds to the nurse's specific knowledge base, enabling them to target health interventions that will avoid exacerbation of health problems such as angina, heart failure, stroke and other arterial diseases.

Respiratory illness

Examples of respiratory disorders experienced as a long-term condition include asthma, cystic fibrosis and chronic obstructive pulmonary disease (COPD – includes bronchitis and emphysema). In the UK around eight million people (about one in seven) – and rising – are affected by a respiratory disease; it is the second most common cause of death. Respiratory illness tends to be more common and more severe in people from lower socio-economic groups; it costs the UK economy nearly £7 billion each year. Smoking is one of a number of causative factors. Adult-trained community nurses frequently manage the care of people with respiratory disease, making detailed assessments of respiratory function, using equipment to monitor respiratory status, prescribing medication and advising on lifestyle and independent living.

Disorders of the nervous system

Common long-term conditions affecting the nervous system (with incidence in UK population) include epilepsy (400,000), multiple sclerosis (60,000), Parkinson's disease (120,000) and cerebral palsy (110,000). Such patients often receive care services managed and delivered by adult nurses in the community, including specialist and advanced practitioners. An example of a specialist adult nurse is a motor neurone disease (MND) nurse. (MND is a progressive neurodegenerative disease that leads to muscle weakness/wasting and increasing loss of limb movement, and difficulties with speech, swallowing and breathing.) MND nurses regularly assess patients in their own homes or a clinic and are then able to use their judgement to help co-ordinate care and specialist rehabilitation services in order to address symptoms. In addition, they support patient groups, families and carers. As with many adult nurses who support people with a long-term condition, MND nurses work interprofessionally to enable their patients to remain at home and live independently as long as possible. The multidisciplinary team in MND typically includes adult nurses, social workers, speech and language therapists, housing advisers, dietitians/nutritionists, physiotherapists, occupational therapists, psychologists and carers.

Diabetes

There are approximately two million people in the UK diagnosed with diabetes plus an estimated one million not yet diagnosed; these figures are increasing annually as a result of an ageing population, decreasing activity levels and increasing weight. Incidence is about 20% for people of South Asian and African-Caribbean communities. Diabetes, especially if not well controlled, significantly increases the risk of: coronary heart disease and stroke; retinopathy (can lead to blindness); neuropathy (damage to small nerves); and peripheral vascular disease (leg ulcers and other damage). Adult nurses are at the forefront of care for people with diabetes and they work with patients as practice nurses, community nurses/matrons, diabetes or wound care (ulcer) specialists; many services are nurse led. Nurse assessment includes not only monitoring blood glucose (sugar) levels and regularly checking for signs of the above complications, but also education, as ultimately it is the way the patient manages their own care every day that has the biggest impact. Providing one-to-one education in a way appropriate for the individual can be challenging and needs to convey an understanding of: the safe use of medicines (e.g. self-administration of insulin); the purpose of insulin and glucose in the body; nutrition and detailed food advice; how to look for problems and what to do; healthy lifestyle opportunities.

Musculo-skeletal system

Most musculo-skeletal health problems are long-term conditions, and many patients experience periods of stability followed by acute exacerbation. Most common are osteo-arthritis (10 million in the UK), rheumatoid arthritis (400,000), osteoporosis (one million) and spinal injuries (paralysis). Specialist (adult) rheumatology nurses are often involved in managing patient care by assessing and monitoring symptoms; examining joints; arranging or reviewing blood tests and other investigations; prescribing/changing treatments; providing information and helping patients learn about their condition; planning care; and making referrals to and receiving referrals from other members of the multidisciplinary team.

Other significant disorders

Other major groups of long-term conditions which adult trained nurses may encounter regularly are skin conditions such as psoriasis, and chronic renal failure.

INTERPROFESSIONAL TEAMS

As adult nurses deliver care in hospitals, other institutions and the community, so their range of work locations is diverse. It is common to find adult nurses working in:

- acute and general hospital wards

- community hospitals

- other state, independent or charity-led institutions

- critical care services such as intensive care or trauma centres

- outpatient and day services

- operating theatres: recovery, 'scrub nurses', surgical assistants

- military health services at home and on posting

- independent sector: hospitals

- independent sectors providing community, on-call or domiciliary care

- practice nursing.

Adult nurses are registered and accountable practitioners, taking personal responsibility for their professional practice and often working autonomously. Whether working independently or in a team, and regardless of where they are working, almost all adult nurses are practising as part of an interprofessional or multidisciplinary team; the importance of a collaborative approach has been widely recognised by the profession and repeatedly in government policy and case inquiries. Interprofessional learning is a strong component of all good nurse training courses.

Son, 63, helping to look after his mum.

case
STUDY

My mum is now 85 years old and, being completely honest, when you see her sat down she easily looks 20 years younger; she looks really well. The trouble is that my mum cannot stand up, as she has both osteoporosis and osteo-arthritis. Technically this is bad news, as it means her bones are weak and might break, and her joints are painful, sometimes swollen and don't really bend much. This is why she is in a chair or wheelchair during the day as she is unable to weight bear (stand on her own legs). She also has very bad arthritis in her hands – the fingers don't move much and her thumbs are locked in one (bad) position. All this seems like it would make someone really down, but not my mum!

Her difficulty is that there are quite a few things she can no longer do for herself; for example, she cannot get into/out of bed, on/off the toilet, cannot walk. Neither can she wash herself, clean herself after using the toilet, do the washing up or cooking, nor can she cut up food. After a short hospital admission to get on top of the pain in her knees, mum was assessed by a community matron [adult nurse] and a social worker; I was there as well as my sister who lives with mum. We agreed, and mum insisted, that she stayed at home as long as she remained well. My sister, 65 years old herself, was worried that she wouldn't be able to give mum the care she needs, so a care package was planned by all of us and mostly paid for by the council.

Mum now has carers come in four times each day to get her up, washed, dressed, toileted during the day and back to bed in the evening. The matron got an occupational therapist to come in with her when the carers started, just to teach them how to use the hoist safely – after all, they need to be careful with my mum. The matron now calls in about once a month and phones once between visits, just to make sure all is well. When she visits there is sometimes a blood test taken; always an examination of mum's knees, hips, elbows and hands; always a check of her pressure areas; she sometimes changes mum's medications, especially her steroids and analgesia [painkillers]. The matron also gets the rheumatology nurse to call in sometimes to give a big injection into mum's shoulder; apparently this is a very skilled job that the matron isn't experienced in.

The interprofessional teams of which adult nurses are a part generally share responsibility for assessing a patient's needs – health and other – planning and delivering care and services together. This requires high standards of communication and flexible working, yet provides the opportunity for a much more holistic or 'whole person' plan of care that avoids duplication (for example of records/notes or assessments). Promoting and delivering cohesive care helps significantly to reduce the impact of physical health difficulties, for example by improving mobility and independence, reducing error by using shared records, understanding and being able to use the expertise of other health professionals. For adult nurses the interprofessional team will be likely to include physiotherapists, psychologists, speech and language therapists, social workers, doctors/surgeons, occupational therapists, housing advisers, podiatrists, benefits advisers, dentists, audiologists, medical scientists, dietitians, education providers, technicians, radiographers and all types of nurses and midwives.

SECTORS IN WHICH ADULT NURSES WORK

It is useful for potential adult nurses to appreciate the range of needs or circumstances some of their patients might face.

Alcohol and substance misuse

Up to 7% of men are alcohol dependent and up to 2% are drug dependent (the figures for women are lower). In addition to risks of mental ill health, users can experience significant, even life-threatening problems with their digestive system, especially the oesophagus and liver. Illness can be distressing and prolonged. Adult nurses working in hospital metabolic and acute medical settings monitor and assess such patients for signs of liver failure (e.g. jaundice/yellow skin and swollen legs), digestive failures and oesophageal bleeding, which can be dramatic and life threatening. In addition, there are key roles as part of the interprofessional team, working alongside medical staff, mental health nurses and counsellors.

Intensive care

Most district and all tertiary hospitals have intensive care units (ICU or ITU); these vary in size but in specialist centres they may be very large, or there may be several of them. In intensive care patients are intensively supported with complex life support and monitoring equipment to (often artificially) maintain respiration, cardiac function and renal function; patients are cared for by experienced adult nurses on a one-to-one basis 24 hours a day. In addition to being able to use technical equipment and administer complex medications, nurses must also ensure high standards of personal care and dignity, liaise with patients' families, ensure that communication with the patient continues and work closely with many other health professionals. Decisions about care often need to be made very quickly and intuition is a key skill. ICU is also one of the few environments where care is the same day and night.

Trauma and orthopaedics

Trauma units typically consist of an accident and emergency department (A&E), an emergency admissions ward and orthopaedic wards supporting people who have had emergency or elective (planned) surgery on bones or joints. The pace of activity in A&E can vary dramatically, and you can be dealing with anything from routine cuts and sprains to major burns, cardiac arrest and haemorrhage. Adult nursing care is inevitably varied and change can be unpredictable – you need to think quickly. Roles can include nurse-led assessment (triage); cleaning wounds; suturing (stitches); taking or ordering blood tests, ECGs and other investigations; prescribing medication. In addition to managing the care needed, nurses also have responsibilities for the related needs of patient and family – anxiety, fear, loss, grieving. Surgery from orthopaedic wards may be urgent, perhaps after bone trauma/fractures, or elective, for example joint replacement.

Women's health

Women's health services typically include treatment for and care of women with breast cancer and reproductive health problems including cancer, uterine fibroids, assisted conception, pre-eclampsia, endometriosis, ovarian cysts and pregnancy. Patients may be young – teenagers. Because of the nature of the illnesses, nurses seek to pay particular attention to emotional health.

Nursing homes

Nursing homes are centres for nursing rather than the media image of 'old people's homes'. Care is led and managed by nurses who use their professional judgement to enable people to improve, maintain or regain health, or to achieve the best possible quality at the end of their life; and nurses work closely with the patients, families, other staff and professionals. Patients may be young and disabled (e.g. have motor neurone disease or be paralysed) or older and physically frail. A key role for adult nurses is to continually assess the needs of patients, then to make detailed plans of care, much of which will be delivered by other care staff whom the adult nurse will supervise. Additionally, there is complex medication to administer, dressings and other treatments to give; and the nurse must at all times be aware of the need to safeguard the vulnerable people in their care. Some nursing homes specialise in caring for people with dementia; these are fully or partly staffed by mental health nurses.

Other areas

Some of the many additional areas of mainly hospital practice where adult nurses work, facilities for which may be found in some general hospitals and most tertiary centres, include: older persons; rehabilitation; burns and plastic surgery; specialist surgery; transplantation; liver/hepatic medicine; travel medicine; dermatology; facio-maxilliary; ear, nose and throat; ophthalmology; infectious diseases; tropical medicine.

ADULT NURSING: THE COURSE

University education is half of the course leading to registration as an adult nurse, and includes areas of study such as:

- professional and ethical practices

- ethical and legal responsibilities

- communication strategies, including for the very vulnerable

- advocacy for clients and their families

- safeguarding

- safe administration of medication

- personal and professional accountability

- political, economic and societal context of care

- delivering care to clients of all ages and in all settings:

  - assessment, planning and evaluation strategies and practices

  - promoting positive physical health messages and behaviours

- ☐ life and social sciences
- ☐ end of life care
- ☐ long-term conditions
- ☐ urgent and unscheduled care
- ☐ pharmacology
- ☐ development of clinical care skills
- ■ managing and leading care:
  - ☐ use of care pathways
  - ☐ interprofessional working
  - ☐ advising and educating patients and other professionals
  - ☐ decision making and clinical leadership
  - ☐ identifying relevant up-to-date evidence for care, and developing and adjusting practices accordingly
  - ☐ anticipating changes in health and 'triggers'
  - ☐ innovative and challenging care in response to patient need.

In all nursing courses, the 'other half' of the course is placement, with a range of opportunities arranged by your university and their health care partners for you to gain insight into and experience of the depth and breadth of adult nursing provision in the local area. Experiences will vary – they will not be the same for all students. Included will be a wide range of clinical need, including: medical and surgical settings; high dependency; urgent/unscheduled/critical care; community care; older persons; ambulatory/non-urgent/outpatient; long-term conditions. Later in the course it is common to have a period of 'client attachment' in the community: in this phase you take increasing responsibility (while supervised) for a group of patients. Students will gain experience where their clients are. This might be in hospital settings (NHS/state or independent hospitals), in the community or in other areas where adults are nursed, for example a nursing home. Students can expect to be supervised and mentored mostly by experienced adult nurses, occasionally by other registered health professionals.

Charlotte is a nursing student in her final year.

Nursing runs in my family: before my sister and myself, my mother and grandmother both had long careers in nursing. This, however, was not my reason for coming into nursing, although it probably influenced my choice. Unlike my sister, I hadn't always wanted to be a nurse. She decided at 7 years old that nursing was what she wanted to do; she is now in her second year of nurse training and is going to make a brilliant nurse. She will also make a different nurse from me. Nurses are all kinds of people, from various walks of life, there isn't an ideal nurse, we are not cloned human beings, a lot of us are not the 'angels' that some people make us out to be, but most of us have a shared purpose, an aim to improve or sustain a person's quality of life.

I came into nursing after falling into a job, purely by chance (or fate), with my local council. I worked as a home care support worker, out in the community, helping people in their homes. I supported service users with nutrition, medication and personal care needs; I did their shopping and cleaning and just had a good chat with them. I met some wonderful people and have continued to meet wonderful people throughout my training. My work as a home care support worker brought a realisation of the pleasure and reward that caring for a person can bring. It was these things that fuelled my desire to become a nurse.

ESSENTIAL SKILLS

When you apply for adult nurse training, selection involves both the university you apply to and their health care practice colleagues. They are looking for a range of skills suitable not just for a three-year degree/

training programme but also for the work you will be doing after you qualify. You might find it useful to begin to highlight your own personal qualities, perhaps in a journal.

The following are essential attributes recognised by nurses:

- excellent and sensitive verbal and non-verbal communication skills with all ages and all groups in society

- a genuine desire to be involved in personal care without prejudice or objection to unpleasant circumstances

- a genuine and non-judgemental interest in all people

- a caring and affable personality

- excellent and dependable communication skills with staff colleagues from many professions, disciplines and sectors

- the ability to engage sensitively with clients of all backgrounds, cultures and beliefs and to learn (assess) from them

- maintaining confidentiality of information, including to/from/between family members

- the potential to learn how to break bad news

- confidence in talking with adults, including people you don't know

- the ability to use intuition, recognising boundaries and limitations

- as training progresses, the ability to learn how to make decisions

- the potential to cope with difficult social situations

- the ability to observe details, especially even minor changes from the 'norm'

- consistency and reliability; a professional approach

- personal integrity

- physical and emotional stamina.

WHY ADULT NURSING?

We have learned that adult nurses have a breathtaking range of roles and responsibilities and have opportunities to work in an incredibly diverse range of settings. It is this diversity and opportunity to change roles, to develop and progress, whilst still having responsibility for patients, that is perhaps the key highlight of adult nursing. It is highly recommended!

Chapter Four
CHILDREN'S NURSING

WHAT DO CHILDREN'S NURSES DO?

Children's nurses deliver professional nursing care to children from birth, including premature birth, to teenagers aged 16 or 18, depending on local arrangements. This modest span of years includes caring for the very diverse health needs of the developing child.

Becky is a premature baby.

case STUDY

Becky was born 13 weeks early and weighed just over 1kg, a little more than a standard bag of sugar. Whilst Becky's physiological structures and systems are fully developed and functioning, some, particularly the lungs, are not yet matured enough for her to live without intensive support. Becky is cared for in a neonatal intensive care unit (NICU), a specialist centre for the most seriously ill babies. In NICU, Becky has one-to-one care from a children's nurse 24 hours a day: the nurse is responsible not just for the physical care of Becky but also for her life support systems. She is nursed in an incubator under phototherapy lamps (to counter jaundice – she is not yet mature enough to synthesise bilirubin) and attached to a ventilator (this machine breathes for Becky as her lungs are immature); heart monitor; temperature probe (premature babies find it difficult to regulate their body temperature); blood oxygen sensor; gastric tube; and two intravenous lines ('drips' to deliver fluids and drugs).

This aspect of children's nursing is very technical; but it is also important to remember that the same nurses are also supporting the parents, who now find themselves feeling rather helpless and bewildered, somewhat cut off from Becky and surrounded by machines with alarms that go off regularly. Infants such as Becky are cared for by a multiprofessional team of health specialists, with care led and managed by children's nurses who have undertaken further training to become advanced neonatal nurse practitioners. It is likely that by the time Becky is 4 months old, about a month after she was expected to be born, she will be able to go home well. About 90% of such premature infants live healthy lives, with no ill effects from their difficult first weeks.

A key factor in successfully nursing children and supporting their families is communication. Most adults, even if they are unwell, are able to describe how they are feeling physically – for example describing a pain or explaining what happened – and to express their concerns – for example their mood or their fear of dying. For younger children especially, the skills of communication – language and relationships – are less developed and lack detail; for example, children with less mature language skills may not be able to distinguish between pain descriptions such as 'aching', 'itching', 'irritating', 'intermittent', 'constant', 'at rest or on movement', 'griping', 'crushing' … and there are many more! The skills learned in children's nurse training include strategies and techniques to identify, assess and interpret a child's behaviours and make rapid decisions based on the evidence the nurse sees.

Tia is a young child with heart problems.

case STUDY

Tia is 3 years old and has several older sisters.
In her infant checkups Tia was noted to have a heart murmur
and a congenital heart defect (structural abnormality in the
heart, present from birth) but recently, when playing with
her older sisters, has become increasingly breathless, often
needing to rest for prolonged periods after exercise. Tia has
now been admitted to a children's cardiac unit for surgery to
repair a hole in the septum (wall) between her two ventricles;
the surgery involves putting Tia on a heart/lung machine
to bypass her own heart while the operation is performed.
Children such as Tia are cared by a diverse multidisciplinary
team working collaboratively. The team can include:

- children's nurses in outpatients, heart ward and intensive care
- theatre nurses (often adult trained)
- doctors, including cardiologists, surgeons, anaesthetist, ICU consultant
- radiographer
- perfusionist
- transfusion team
- theatre and ICU technicians
- biochemist
- and many more!

The children's nurses involved have experience and training
in extended skills. The enables them to deliver skilled practice
and lead decision making linked to assessment, technical
treatment and ongoing holistic care of Tia and her family.
Nursing care can include:

- the use of complex life support equipment
- determining and administering correct medications
- assessment and monitoring of Tia's condition

- helping Tia and her parents re-establish independence in personal care
- supporting Tia, her sisters and parents in a family-centred approach.

In addition, there is a wide range of essential processes to monitor and support Tia, involving the children's nurse regularly assessing vital signs such as blood pressure, heart rate, respiratory function, temperature (for signs of infection), urine output/fluid intake (kidney function), restoration of diet/digestive functions and education support to avoid future adverse events such as endocarditis (infection in the heart).

As you can see, nursing a child is diverse, and children have not just physical health needs but also emotional, learning, developmental and psychosocial needs. In learning to become a children's nurse students gain a comprehensive insight into:

- the development of a healthy child towards adulthood
- strategies and techniques for clinical practice
- helping minimise the impact of illness, health impairment or hospital admission on the child.

This always involves working in partnership with many other health professionals, parents and family, or whoever looks after the child at home. It is common for the children's nurse to be a lead practitioner in both hospital and community settings.

CHILDREN'S NURSES WITHIN THE HEALTH CARE SYSTEM

Traditionally, a common perception has been that unwell children are cared for in hospital settings, the place of employment for many children's nurses. Now, however, many children are cared for entirely outside of hospital – for many good reasons:

**Alice (22) is in her final year
of child nursing training.**

case
STUDY

During my three years at university I spent half of
my placements within the community setting, working with
a range of different professionals who come into contact
with children and their families. It is fantastic to get involved
with health visitors, going on visits to check newborn babies,
working through to a 2-year check; as well as supporting
postnatally depressed mums and children deemed at risk.
I was fortunate enough to spend two weeks with a school
nurse based in a setting for children with physical disabilities
and complex medical needs; this was a fantastic experience,
getting to work alongside many other professionals and even
helping the children in a swimming lesson! With the community
nurses I experienced visits with the diabetes nurse specialist
and routine assessments with children with a chronic illness.
This interested and captivated me so much that I am now
writing my dissertation on how parents and siblings adjust to
chronic illness in the family.

- it enables the child to live in their own home and maintain family and
  peer relationships

- there is a lower risk of acquiring infection, which is particularly
  important for those receiving treatment for cancer

- it helps avoid rapidly learned dependence on hospital staff

- it is more cost-effective

- it allows the family to continue to provide personal care, something
  many people find awkward in hospitals

- it is less stressful for the child, and helps them maintain some control
  over their care.

With more and more children receiving health care outside hospitals, the
work locations for children's nurses are also changing, with an increasing

number working in the community, schools, children's centres, hospices and a wide range of specialist and charity settings.

Tom is 3 years old and has Down's syndrome.

case STUDY

As well as the easily recognised facial features, dribbling and pronounced enlarged tongue, Tom has also had a surgical repair to a small congenital heart defect associated with his syndrome. Tom also has impaired cognition, with delayed walking (since just before his 3rd birthday); his speech is limited to a handful of words and he seems clumsy, having difficulty in feeding himself and playing with certain toys. Tom is cared for by his parents and older sisters, who are highly committed to helping him. He is also supported by a range of professionals including a health visitor, community-based children's nurse, speech and language therapist and a weekly play scheme for children with his range of needs. One of the key roles of the children's nurse is to assess Tom and act as an information conduit, linking parental needs and anxieties, Tom's assessments and the opportunities and care available from others involved in his care. A key aim is to keep Tom well and avoid hospital admissions for commonly associated conditions such as constipation and chest infection/pneumonia.

AREAS OF SUPPORT FROM CHILDREN'S NURSES

The mass media portrayal of children's nursing often paints a picture of active children, playrooms with the latest electronic toys, celebrity visitors and relaxed but hardworking nurses. Of course, we are all well aware that reality is often rather different from such images and it is important for potential children's nurses to appreciate the range of needs and difficulties their patients might face. These might include the following.

Megan is 17 and has diabetes, diagnosed when she was 6 years old.

case STUDY

Megan self-cares – in other words, she tests her own blood sugar levels and administers her own insulin injections every day, varying the dose depending on the blood test result. Megan's school is well aware of her diabetes, largely because a specialist paediatric diabetic community nurse has been supporting her (and her parents). The role of the nurse has largely been to educate Megan:

- explaining and exploring with her how insulin is needed in the body
- what happens when production fails (as in diabetes)
- safe blood testing and injecting
- the significance of puberty, growth and exercise.

Now the nurse is preparing Megan for 'transition' – the phase of care where the young person begins to move from child health services to adult services. This transition can be important, as this stage of life is full of distractions, emotional development and the beginnings of an adult lifestyle. The nurse works with Megan, her family, school and college to ensure high levels of understanding and that Megan continues to be compliant with her care. The nurse's aim is to keep Megan independent, and Megan has not required any hospital admissions to date.

Premature birth babies

About 90% of children born three months prematurely survive with no lasting effects, but 10% will not survive or will have long-term needs/ disability. Such children often need very intensive support for many months. Children's nurses working in such environments (see Becky's story on page 45) can find themselves drawn into the trauma the family face and, in addition to the 'hands on' care of the infant and technical challenges, there are very high levels of responsibility and emotional involvement. In such an environment nurses must also be prepared for the child to not survive, and to support family members and colleagues through the inevitable grief that follows.

Teenagers

As 'nearly adults', teenagers often suffer adult-type trauma – crashing cycles, rugby injuries, substance misuse – which can result in major neurological damage, broken bones, etc. While the majority recover fully, others suffer long-term disability or loss of independence. Nursing care inevitably varies according to need, but it can include:

- observations of cardiovascular, respiratory, renal and temperature status, function and viability of injured limbs

- working with physiotherapists to advance rehabilitation

- working with parents/family to enable them to get involved in giving care and promoting independence

- careful administration of medication such as analgesia, often on a per kg of body weight basis

- liaison with school/school nurses

- age-appropriate education for the patient and/or family for self-care after discharge home.

Diabetes/epilepsy/arthritis/asthma

These long-term conditions can affect children at any age. Care is often very successfully managed by the patient/family and/or community nurses. Acute exacerbations can happen requiring urgent hospital intervention; a small number of deaths occur each year. Children with the more common long-term conditions frequently have a specialist children's nurse as their lead health specialist. For example, a paediatric diabetes nurse specialises in the holistic care of a child with diabetes from infancy through to adolescence, developing, implementing and evaluating programmes of care and providing specialist clinical advice to health carers, family, schools and others. Working from a hospital or community base (or both), the nurses:

- advise on management of diabetes including diet, medication and complications

- give one-to-one teaching for the child, family and others, particularly promoting safe self-care and giving a strong knowledge base

- give counselling

- advise on lifestyle and long-term health issues

- undertake nurse-led clinics, including clinical assessment and blood testing

- adjust insulin type and dose

- interpret and act on specialist investigations

- safeguard the children in their care.

Diarrhoea/vomiting

Young children, especially infants, have limited reserves of fluid and nutrients. Continued diarrhoea and/or vomiting can rapidly cause the child to become dehydrated; they will be admitted to hospital for intravenous fluids. In hospital the children's nurse will prioritise the safety of the child, and procedures will include frequent and accurate assessment of cardiac, respiratory and renal function, neurological status, skin and temperature. Dehydration is a serious risk, potentially damaging the kidneys and other vital organs; pyrexia (above-normal body temperature) can become uncontrolled, leading to neurological/brain damage. The care needed includes urgent and very accurate administration of drugs to reduce temperature, other cooling strategies and careful intravenous rehydration – all this in an infant likely to be very frightened, not responding normally and with a very anxious parent accompanying. What is perhaps a 'routine illness' becomes a key ground for high-quality nursing care and family engagement, with discharge likely within 48 hours.

Cancer

We are often reluctant to accept that children get cancer. Survival rates for some cancers have improved dramatically but at the moment, perhaps after years of treatment, the outcome may still be death in childhood. There are a number of roles for children's nurses, including nurses in cancer care units, where their specialist roles include administration of complex chemotherapy drugs, other treatments, monitoring vital signs, reducing side effects of medication, and strategies to avoid secondary infection, such as nursing the child in isolation facilities. A child may well be known to the hospital nurse team for a year or more, and close relationships can develop; these are often vital for the child and family but can be personally challenging for the nurse. Children's nurses also work in palliative (end of life) care in both hospice settings and the child's own home; these nurses also need psychological skills to support bereaved siblings and families and the ability to make rational professional decisions in the most trying of circumstances.

Congenital/from birth conditions

Advances in care for unwell/premature babies has led to an increased survival rate of children with congenital problems. Defects might be obvious from birth or later and can be very rare (e.g. conjoined twins) or more common (e.g. cleft palate or Downs syndrome). Children often have complex and unique needs. There are a multitude of health care interventions, determined by need, with children's nurses providing nursing care in hospital medical and surgical units, as well as in the community. An additional role is that of the paediatric genetics adviser – a children's nurse specialising in supporting both child and family through the complicated world of genetics. This involves working with the family to trace familial histories and making a detailed assessment of the child to ascertain a precise diagnosis, which will enable the adviser to give detailed genetics advice, predict health needs and make plans for early interventions or prevention.

Learning/developmental problems

Developmental disabilities cause significant difficulty with communication (including speech) and social interactions (behaviours). Symptoms can arise in the first year, diagnosis is usually made by the age of 3; delay in many learned skills from infancy onwards is typical. This category includes children with autistic spectrum disorders (including Asperger's syndrome), sensory disabilities and some metabolic disorders. Typically, nurses help lead multi-agency care in community (e.g. Sure Start) or home settings with extensive advocacy for the child/family and liaison with a very diverse range of health, social and education professionals. The interprofessional team will be likely to include, in addition to the well-established health professionals, play therapists, psychologists, social workers, dietitians, infant hearing screeners and health visitors.

Parents/family

Most children are supported by parents or family members who care deeply about their unwell child but are very anxious and often feel disempowered by the health services they experience. A key role of all children's nurses is to ensure care is family centred, with parents well informed and participating in care.

CHILDREN'S NURSING: THE COURSE

University education is half of the course leading to registration as a children's nurse, and includes areas of study such as:

- professional and ethical practices
- ethical and legal responsibilities, including all safeguarding legislation
- communication strategies: children, families and community
- advocacy for clients and their families
- safe administration of medication
- working to support individual rights; anti-discrimination
- political, economic and societal context of care
- delivering care to children from birth to adolescence/teenagers and in all settings through:
    - ☐ assessment strategies and practices
    - ☐ promoting positive health messages and behaviours
    - ☐ educating children, their families and significant others
    - ☐ life and social sciences
    - ☐ pharmacology
    - ☐ life support and end of life care skills
    - ☐ clinical care skills/technical skills

- managing and leading care through:
    - [ ] co-ordinating care on an interprofessional basis
    - [ ] decision making and clinical leadership
    - [ ] identifying relevant up-to-date evidence for nursing children, developing and adjusting practices accordingly
    - [ ] anticipating physical and emotional changes
    - [ ] innovative and challenging care in response to clients' and families' needs.

As in all other nursing courses, the other half of a children's nursing course is placement. You will experience a range of opportunities arranged for you, in which you will gain insight into and experience of the diversity of children's health and nursing care. Experiences will vary according to specific universities and health trusts, but they will always include a wide range of ages (including neonatal/toddler to adolescent/teenagers) and dependences (may range from school nursing and health visiting to children's trauma unit, hospice, intensive care or specialist neurological or cardiac centre). It is normal to have several placement experiences in community settings, reflecting the gradual shift in children's health care away from acute hospitals. Students can expect to be supervised and mentored mostly by experienced children's nurses, and occasionally by other registered health professionals.

ESSENTIAL SKILLS

Applying for a place to train as a children's nurse is a particularly competitive process, involving both the university you apply to and their child health practice colleagues. They are looking for a range of skills suitable not only for a three-year degree/training programme but also for the work you will be doing as a child nurse after you qualify. You might find it useful to begin to highlight your own qualities, perhaps in a journal.

The following are essential attributes recognised by nurses:

- excellent and sensitive verbal and non-verbal communication skills with children

Stephanie (20) is a child nursing student.

case STUDY

When I left school I wasn't entirely sure what I wanted my career to be so I chose to study the CACHE Diploma in Childcare and Education Studies alongside an A level in Drama. When looking at university courses, based on my course experiences I decided to commit to nursing as I would get to work alongside children and make a difference to people's lives. Although it has been hard work, I am so glad I made the decision to study children's nursing as I have thoroughly enjoyed working with children and families from a range of backgrounds and with a variety of care needs, as well as developing my interprofessional working skills. The highlight of my course so far has been a module exploring urgent and unscheduled care, as it was brilliant to develop my knowledge and skills within this area, particularly extending my understanding of safeguarding vulnerable groups. As part of the assessment for this module I also undertook an emergency situation skills session and as part of a small group worked with a 'real' (simulator that breathes and responds in real time) child whilst having instructions from professionals and additional incidents taking place. Although at the time this was a daunting experience, it was great to experience the emergency environment in safe hands and subsequently reflect on the session with a lecturer.

- excellent and consistent communication skills with adults such as parents and colleagues from many professions

- the ability to play sensitively with children and to learn (assess) from this

- recognition of the importance of confidentiality of information, including to/from/between family members

- the ability to learn how to respond to distressed adults/parents

- confidence in talking with adults (e.g. for teaching parents)

- the ability to use intuition and recognise boundaries

- feeling comfortable about dealing with personal care and body fluids (e.g. blood, urine)

- the ability to observe small details, especially changes from the 'norm'

- consistency and reliability

- a professional approach

- personal integrity.

WHY CHILDREN'S NURSING?

This chapter has explored just some of the diversity of roles that children's nurses undertake and the range of settings they can work in. Although there might be some similarities to adult nursing, there are few professions that have such a range of 'clients', from premature infants through to the cusp of adulthood. It is also important to remember the changing context of children's nursing: with hospital stays becoming shorter, the associated nursing care is more acute and interventional. Yet, in the community, there is a steady expansion of roles so that many children previously nursed in a hospital or institution now receive complex and advanced nursing care in their own home or even at school. If you have compassion for and understanding of children **and** their families, together with an inner resolve to make difficult decisions, children's nursing might well be for you – do consider it!

Chapter Five
MENTAL HEALTH NURSING

WHAT DO MENTAL HEALTH NURSES DO?

It is estimated that in Western Europe, mental health problems and treatable mental illness will affect at least 20% of the adult population at some stage of their life and up to 10% of children aged under 16. Mental health nurses are the lead health professionals in this field of practice, and their training equips them to treat and support people with mental health needs.

One of the very important points to realise when considering mental health nursing is that the people mental health nurses support are unwell. We are all familiar with people we know having a physical illness; in fact it is often a talking point, with questions often being asked and answered freely, scars shown, medication discussed, plaster casts signed and so on. However, it is much less common to share similarly intimate conversation about anxieties we have, our low mood or our treatment for psychoses or behavioural difficulties. Such exchanges rarely happen, and when they do we are often uncertain how to respond. Of course, mental illness is just that – an illness – for which the patient needs support and treatment with an array of possible therapies in order to recover or live optimally with a long-term condition.

Preparation for becoming a mental health nurse includes promotion of mental health wellbeing and prevention of mental ill health as well as developing expertise in therapeutic intervention for those experiencing mental illness. As in all areas of nursing, studying includes physiology

Emma, 25, is a mental health nurse specialising in bereavement and loss.

Emma found life difficult when she was growing up. There was an older sister who was always out, an older brother who picked on her, and mum. Mum was always there, in Emma's face, arguing with her, blaming her for absolutely everything, shouting at her in front of grandparents and neighbours. Occasionally mum was nice, but she was often angry, and much more interested in herself than in Emma. At 14 Emma ran away, not far – and with no money she had to go home to be shouted at and punished. Emma rebelled privately; she didn't eat: when her mum made her eat, she would vomit later; her weight began to drop dramatically. By 15 Emma was ill, obsessed by not eating; still lonely and feeling unwanted, she tried to harm herself. At this point, assessed by both a GP and a psychiatrist, Emma was admitted to an adolescent mental health unit, a nurse-led unit, and she found that the nurses were great – they genuinely cared for her and wanted her better. After two months of counselling and cognitive behavioural therapy Emma was discharged to live with her aunt with continuing assessment by the same Child and Adolescent Mental Health Service (CAMHS) mental health nurses. Friends noticed the profound change in Emma, both in her physical health and in her attitude. Determined to pay back what she had received, Emma completed GCSEs, achieving reasonable results, then took a health and social care course at sixth-form college. Now successfully trained and registered as a mental health nurse, Emma is employed by a charity working with people who have been recently bereaved.

and life sciences, social sciences such as psychology, sociology and behavioural science, as well as communication, pharmacology and health services.

Sean, aged 28, is a manager of a large supermarket.

Sean regarded himself as a normal child but perhaps quieter than his peers, with few friends and largely being self-occupied. When Sean got his job as a trainee manager he moved away from home into a company shared house, and it was here, with new acquaintances, that he began to use marijuana regularly and experiment with cocaine most weekends. Of course, the company found out, Sean was sacked, and he was forced to move back home, becoming markedly depressed, unable to sleep or even rest, with what he calls 'a black hole' of unpleasant thoughts and feelings about losing his job and 'being caught'. Parental pressure eventually led him to go to the family doctor and, after medications proved unsuccessful, Sean was admitted to a local mental health hospital.

Here he spent time talking with the nursing team and eventually a diagnosis of schizophrenia was made. Daily medication stopped Sean having his 'black thoughts' and lifted his depression, but he was frightened at the 'label' of schizophrenia because the media associate schizophrenia with violent and frightening crime. Finding it difficult to trust what he read or what his parents told him, Sean was encouraged to continue taking his medications by his community mental health nurse, with whom a trusting relationship has developed. The nurse continues to see Sean every other month and phones him in between times; if Sean has a difficult day or feels his symptoms are returning he is able to telephone the community nursing team for advice or adjustment to treatment, any day until 8.00 p.m. After five at least partially lost years, Sean has now successfully trained as a manager with a different company, working full time; his employers are fully supportive of his long-term health status.

Until the 1980s, in the UK at least, people with mental health disorders were normally cared for in institutions, often hospitals some distance from towns and cities. This system, essentially carried forward (with much improvement) from the asylums of Victorian times, was heavily criticised for being impersonal, inhibiting choice and restricting families, employment opportunities and social engagement. Since then, there has been much progress in introducing and delivering community care, which aims to support and care for people in their own homes wherever possible, rather than provide care in an a institution or residential establishment. In addition to the freedom, human rights and moral improvements, community care has also been demonstrated to be less expensive and the standards of care much higher. A further benefit of community-focused care has been to redefine the relationship between social care and health care provision and to encourage partnerships in care between state health care providers (e.g. the NHS), local authorities/social services, the private sector and charitable organisations (e.g. MIND).

Saeeda, aged 24, is a housewife.

case STUDY

Like her parents, Saeeda was born in the UK, though her appearance is clearly like that of her Bangladeshi grandparents. It was only at secondary school that other children began to make what she now calls racist comments about how she looked – her skin colour was obviously different – despite her clear regional accent! Saeeda's family realised what was going on and were worried for their daughter. They tried to help protect her from the comments by busying her in the family store and with family gatherings.

Before long it became clear to Saeeda that she wasn't the only one at her school who was subject to racist bullying; in fact it seemed that the white majority seemed to gang together in making school life intolerable for the several Asian and Afro-Caribbean pupils. Even tutor group 'friends' joined in the antagonism. Saeeda felt two things: first, she felt great loneliness and second, she was very cross, very angry – she hated what she was experiencing and those behind it. It was this that led her into joining a teenage gang, a group that at the time seemed to tick all the right boxes – they hated being pushed around and insulted because of their skin colour. After several fights, a visit to hospital with a cut wrist resulting from a fight and the involvement of the school authorities, Saeeda recognised she was at a critical point and agreed to be referred to CAMHS.

Following a number of visits for assessment, the mental health nurse engaged Saeeda in a programme of cognitive behavioural therapy and helped her to explore a series of goals; learning and practising new skills and approaches to help meet these goals is often successful. Saeeda continued at the same school, successfully becoming a regular member of the drama team, completing her studies and then stopping her meetings with CAMHS.

MENTAL HEALTH NURSES WITHIN THE HEALTH CARE SYSTEM

The vast majority of people with mental ill health are cared for in the community, either in their own homes or at clinics and day care facilities; consequently, the majority of mental health nurses also work in community settings. Such arrangements allow nurses to offer assessment and therapy, and there are significant advantages to patients and clients:

- it supports independent living, with opportunity for normal family and social relationships

- it helps avoid dependence on institutions and full-time staff

- it avoids the awkwardness of family/friends having to visit an institution

- it is considerably more cost-effective to the state/health service

- it allows the opportunity for employment, education, holidays, own food, social events, etc.

- the patient retains substantial control over the nature and timing of their care.

As mental health nurses deliver ever-increasing amounts of care in the community, so their work locations also change. It is common to find mental health nurses working in:

- prisons/custody centres

- alcohol and/or substance misuse services

- acute admissions wards

- psychiatric intensive care units

- military health services

- older persons' mental health services, e.g. for patients with dementia

- CAMHS, e.g. for patients with eating disorders

- forensic/secure services for adults or children.

Working in such a diversity of settings, especially in the community, mental health nurses are recognised as lead specialists amongst the diverse multidisciplinary teams supporting their clients. Often directing the care delivered by others as well as their own clinical load, mental health nurses are fully accountable registered practitioners. The work is additionally challenging as face-to-face support of clients can often be on a one-to-one basis, without the reassurance of a large team available around the corner.

Interprofessional teams

Promoting and delivering cohesive interprofessional care may significantly reduce mental ill health difficulties, for example by resolving difficult housing situations. For mental health nurses the interprofessional team will be likely to include:

- psychologists

- social workers

Harold was diagnosed with Alzheimer's disease.

Harold was 76 and had not long celebrated his golden wedding anniversary when he began to forget. At first it was little things – he forgot to take letters with him to post, to take change from shopkeepers; and then he forgot his own birthday, being very surprised that he was having a family party. Nobody thought too much of it, friends even teased him that he was getting old. Unfortunately, within a year Harold's 'forgetfulness' was becoming a problem, not just for himself but also for family and acquaintances. Harold would get very cross with his wife, demanding breakfast even though the empty dishes were still in front of him; he would put on his trousers back to front, inevitably frustrated when using the lavatory; and he would scowl at long-standing friends and family who visited, seeming not to know who they were.

Harold was diagnosed with Alzheimer's disease and was prescribed medication, which appeared to slow the loss of memory and unusual behaviour.

Alzheimer's is the most common of many types of dementia, all of which are progressive; the structure and chemistry of the brain become increasingly damaged over time. Referral was also made to the local community psychiatric nurses (CPNs), trained mental health nurses with experience and/or extended training for working in the community. CPNs provide treatment, care and support for people with Alzheimer's and all types of dementia. The CPN assessed Harold in his home, advising both him and his wife on strategies for coping with daily activities, and about improving their general health and wellbeing. Two years after his ill health became apparent, Harold deteriorated, twice getting lost on the short walk home from the local shops, a daily activity for many years; his wife began to find herself exhausted by caring for Harold, not least because regular incontinence meant two laundry loads each day. Harold was admitted to a community mental health hospital as a respite break for his wife and for assessment of his medication. Sadly, Harold passed away shortly afterwards.

- housing advisers

- employment/supported employment services

- benefits advisers

- court services

- occupational therapists

- art/creative therapists

- dietitians, e.g. for eating disorders

- schools and education providers

- hostels

- and all types of nurses and midwives.

Working with such a diverse range of professionals demands meticulous communication and flexibility in working practices, but it is demonstrably more responsive to patient needs, more holistic and, since it avoids duplication of assessment/records, more efficient and less expensive.

AREAS OF SUPPORT FROM MENTAL HEALTH NURSES

The media often draw unhelpful attention to mental ill health, reinforcing the stigma felt by patients. Of course, we are all well aware that the stigma is real, despite the efforts of campaigners and professionals; it is important for potential mental health nurses to appreciate the range of needs and difficulties their patients might face, some of which are listed below.

Helen, aged 26, is a newly qualified mental health nurse.

case STUDY

For me, making the decision to apply for mental health nurse training took a long time. I'd always known that I wanted to work with people, to do something that felt worthwhile and significant. I always thought I would work in the public sector in some capacity, but was unsure of which role I would be best suited to. I went to university first, got a degree in psychology and worked in different public sector settings along the way to help guide me. Voluntary work at a hospital and a stint working in social services and in hospital outpatients all served to inform my decision making.

For me, personal experiences formed a key part of the journey towards mental health nursing. At university, a close friend of mine suffered with mental health problems, but perhaps most significant was my grandmother's experience of dementia and the wider impact that this had on my family. These experiences combined, then helped me to better understand the role of the mental health nurse and to develop a passion for working in this area.

As a student nurse, I particularly enjoyed working with older people with mental health problems and especially people with dementia. It was rewarding in so many ways and often it was the small things that made the biggest difference. Playing old wartime songs to a distressed patient and watching them settle and begin to sing along, helping a confused patient to find their handbag, assisting a patient with poor sequencing skills to get washed and dressed. These seemingly small acts would often allow a glimmer of the person before dementia to shine through. Alongside these experiences, the challenge and interest of such issues as medication management, physical health care, and assessment and discharge planning made working in this environment feel worthwhile, dynamic and interesting.

Nurse training has been one of the toughest things I've done. It has been challenging in so many ways, but I wouldn't change it. Stepping into the world of mental health nursing has afforded me such a privilege; I get to help people through what can be the most difficult times in their life.

Alcohol and substance misuse

Up to 7% of men are alcohol dependent and up to 2% are drug dependent (figures for women are lower). Mental ill health, e.g. depression or anxiety, is common and each either leads to or underpins the other: alcohol, itself a depressant, compounds the problem and over-use may lead to dependence.

Mental health nurses often lead client care, using, for example, cognitive therapy or psychotherapies. The caring relationship may be in an NHS/state, charitable or private health setting, but is likely to continue for an extended period of time. Nurses need the ability and resolve to support their clients through both success and failure.

Children/teenagers

Mental health problems affect up to 10% of children aged under 16; a small number experience severe illness. Illnesses can include behavioural problems such as sleep and/or soiling/wetting difficulty, and can be exacerbated by the impact of divorce, bereavement, bullying, abuse or trauma. Eating disorders and obsessive–compulsive disorder can appear. Mental health nurses work with children and young people in their own homes, at school, community facilities and in hospitals. Quality, trusting relationships, which can take time to establish, are essential in order to be able to make a detailed assessment and diagnosis prior to planning and delivering therapeutic interventions. Nurses work closely with psychologists, schools, youth offending teams and youth services.

Forensic/secure services

Nurses provide health care for people with mental disorders who are offenders or at risk of offending. Services are provided in secure and community NHS and criminal justice (prison) settings. Patients include difficult, dangerous and/or extremely vulnerable people whose behaviour presents a risk to themselves and others. Nurses engage in assessment, treatment and other therapeutic services in the context of legal, security and public safety protocols. This group of services includes secure services for children and young people. Safe working practices are essential to safeguard patients (from both self-harm and harm by other patients), staff and the public (to de-escalate potential aggression or disorder).

Pregnancy/childbirth

A woman's mental state can impact on the development and/or birth of the foetus or child, and affect the family. Where there is past or present severe mental illness, specialist perinatal mental health services may be involved. Mother and baby units support mental health nursing for women needing in-patient care within 12 months of childbirth. Depression and anxiety are the most frequent illnesses; nurses may engage in cognitive therapies or psychotherapies. Care may also be delivered in community clinics and a client's own home.

Bipolar disorder

This used to be called 'manic depression'; sufferers have very severe mood swings lasting weeks or months, with low (depressive) periods of intense despair and high (manic) periods with an extreme sense of wellbeing, energy and optimism. Bipolar disorder affects about one person in every hundred. In addition to medication, psychological treatments, often nurse led, include mood monitoring, mood strategies and cognitive therapies. As well as formal therapies, mental health nurses support people with bipolar disorder by helping them recognise, then address symptoms as they arise as well as manage the side effects of their medication.

Alzheimer's/dementia

Dementia is a progressive brain disease, often starting with memory problems; there are also difficulties with communication, mood/personality changes, coping with daily tasks. As the disease progresses, so independence diminishes. It can start from around the age of 40 (early onset); about one in 20 people over the age of 65 have dementia, and this rises to one in five of people aged over 80. Alzheimer's disease is the commonest cause. Mental health nurses help the patient and family deal with the complex psychosocial issues, offer counselling and family education, and advise on medication. The role of mental health nurses in supporting this group of clients is recognised by continuing research (Scotland's Mental Health and its Context: Adults, 2009), which particularly emphasises the value of emotional support and advice, liaison and networking, training and education, and – for people in the early stages of dementia – counselling that considers associated language and cognitive deficits.

Other significant disorders

The following are often considered to be major mental health illnesses, potentially suffered by people of all ages to varying degrees of severity:

- phobias

- obsessive compulsive disorder

- personality disorders

- post-traumatic stress disorder

- schizophrenia

- seasonal affective disorder; eating disorders.

MENTAL HEALTH NURSING: THE COURSE

University education is half of the course leading to registration as a mental health nurse, and includes areas of study such as:

- professional and ethical practices

- ethical and legal responsibilities, especially under the Mental Health Act

- communication strategies, including for the very vulnerable

- advocacy for clients and their families

- safeguarding patients, including safe administration of medication

- working to support individual rights and anti-discrimination

- political, economic and societal context of care

- delivering care to clients of all ages and in all settings through:

  ☐ assessment strategies and practices

  ☐ psychosocial interventions

  ☐ promoting positive mental and physical health messages and behaviours

  ☐ life and social sciences

  ☐ pharmacology of mental health drugs

  ☐ development of clinical care skills

- managing and leading care through:

  ☐ co-ordinating care pathways on a multi-agency basis

  ☐ advising and educating clients, families and other professionals

  ☐ decision making and clinical leadership

  ☐ identifying relevant up-to-date evidence for mental health care, and developing and adjusting practices accordingly

  ☐ anticipating client behaviour, changes and 'triggers'

  ☐ innovative and challenging care in response to clients' and families' needs.

As in other nursing courses, the other half of the course is placement, with a range of opportunities provided for you to gain insight into and to experience the depth and breadth of mental health nursing provision in the local area. Experiences will vary but will always include a wide range of ages (including child/adolescent and elderly/dementia), dependences (from fully independent in care to full physical and mental dependence) and behaviours, including challenging behaviour, addictions and perhaps forensic or custodial care. It is common to have an extended period of 'client attachment' where, while supervised, you take increasingly independent responsibility for a client over a period of many months. Students will gain experience where their clients are based: sometimes this will be in acute hospital or other institutional settings but it will most frequently be in the community. Work may be with clients being cared for by the NHS or in local authority, prison/police, independent (private) and charitable settings. Students can expect to be supervised and mentored by both experienced mental health nurses and other registered and relevant professionals.

Whilst retaining their independence as registered nurses and accountability for their practice, mental health nurses frequently share responsibility for their clients with an extended multidisciplinary team. These interprofessional teams often share a single client assessment – looking at health, mental, social and other needs – and plan and deliver care or services together. This requires high standards of communication and flexible working, yet gives opportunity for a much more holistic and cost-effective plan of care that avoids duplication. Promoting and delivering such cohesive care also helps avoid gaps and maintains standards in care provision.

Alex, 32, mental health nursing student.

case STUDY

When I was at school I was popular with friends and often on the edge of trouble – I didn't ever 'do' anything but was often in the front row watching! I managed to do quite well, with 7 GCSEs at C or better, then, being rather uninterested in sixth form, just one A level. I wanted to work and have some money, and got a job as a trainee accountant; the money was okay but I liked the weekends, so much so that I was taken home by the police more than once.

It was when I was 26 that my granddad became ill; he couldn't remember things and even forgot who I was sometimes. I would go to his house to try to help – do the shopping, gardening, clean his place through – but was often sad that granddad no longer seemed to be the same person I knew.

I sometimes sat with my mum while the dementia nurse tried to help granddad, talking about the past, making suggestions about how he might use the bathroom more reliably (instead of 'missing') and manage around his home. One day granddad came to our house – we still have no idea how he walked five miles, let alone without getting knocked over. The nurse helped us to talk with granddad and he now lives in a nursing home for people who, like him, have dementia; he misses being outdoors but still appears to enjoy himself; he doesn't seem to know me now but I'm glad that he seems pleased to see anyone!

My experience with granddad made me rethink what I was doing with life; I had really enjoyed helping him instead of just doing things for myself. I got myself a job as a health care assistant at a mental health day centre where many 'patients' reminded me a bit of granddad. The staff said I should be a nurse as I had lots of good qualities to offer; as they were quite insistent I looked into it and now, after passing an Access course to improve on my exams, I am really enjoying my first year of mental health nurse training.

ESSENTIAL SKILLS

Mental ill health is one of the most common health problems. Caring for people with mental ill health is not for everyone: the qualities and patience needed to build effective caring relationships are unique. Universities and health providers look for the attributes of both a successful student and a future mental health nurse. It is not always easy to recognise these skills in ourselves – perhaps nurses are sometimes too humble. Highlighting your own personal qualities, perhaps in a journal, is useful preparation.

The following are essential attributes recognised by nurses:

■ excellent and sensitive verbal and non-verbal communication skills with all ages and all groups in society

■ a genuine interest in all people

- a caring and affable personality

- reliable and consistent listening – this is especially important

- excellent and dependable communication skills with colleagues from many professions, disciplines and sectors

- the ability to engage sensitively with clients of all backgrounds, cultures and beliefs and to learn (assess) from this

- recognition of the importance of confidentiality of information, including to/from/between family members

- the potential to learn how to respond to distressed people and family members

- confidence in talking with adults, including people you don't know

- the ability to use intuition, recognising boundaries and limitations

- as training progresses, the ability to learn how to and then to make decisions

- the potential to cope with difficult or distressing social situations, deprivation, disordered/chaotic homes

- the ability to observe detail, especially even minor changes from the 'norm'

- consistency and reliability

- a professional approach

- personal integrity.

WHY MENTAL HEALTH NURSING?

This chapter explored some of the diversity of mental health nursing roles and briefly highlighted some of the settings in which mental health nurses work. Some practitioners are drawn to mental health nursing because of the range of opportunities and the potential to change from one setting to another; others are attracted by the deep and often enduring caring relationship with clients; for others, it is the intrigue of engaging with the mind – unseen and not always fully understood – that appeals. Whatever your motivation, carefully evaluate your own qualities and go ahead with gaining experience or making your application.

Chapter Six
LEARNING DISABILITIES NURSING

WHAT IS A LEARNING DISABILITY?

In most areas of professional health care there is a fundamental premise of 'trying to fix things', whether the desired result is making the patient better or providing comfort in the end stages of life. For people who have a learning disability, that goal of getting better is not achievable. Instead, professional learning disability nurses offer individual support and intervention to allow development of independence, skills and fulfilment in life.

There is not yet universal agreement on use of the term 'learning disability'. In many countries, developed and developing, other descriptors are used, including 'intellectual disability', 'mental handicap' and 'mental retardation'. In the UK 'learning disability' is almost universally used by health, social and education professionals as well as support groups and the general public.

There is sometimes confusion about just what a learning disability is, yet the term is straightforward – it refers to people of any age whose learning is disabled. Having a learning disability is not the same as having dyslexia, dyscalculia (see page 82) or mental ill health.

This chapter is mainly concerned with exploring the nature of learning disability nursing but will briefly look at the professions supporting people who have a specific learning difficulty.

Gary is 39, has a moderate to severe learning disability and lives with three other people, similar to himself, in a community home – his home.

case
STUDY

Gary's parents looked after him in their family home until 10 years ago, but as they were then 78 and 80 years old, they no longer felt able to manage his care. Gary does need regular input from others – for example being reminded to do most things, such as going to the toilet or to bed and help with showering; he also soils the bed about twice a week. Gary's behaviour follows a regular pattern of being placid until there is even the slightest change in routine; this seems to trigger a lot of anxiety and behaviour which staff find difficult, including rushing around, storming into rooms and often knocking into things on the way. This is an example of challenging behaviour.

The nurses working with Gary started noticing that he began to breathe very noisily, sometimes associated with coughing, when he was asleep. After treatment for a chest infection Gary's breathing settled but staff then noticed a change in behaviour, with periods in which Gary would sit still, apparently 'gazing into space' and appearing disconnected from other people/activities. Over the course of a few weeks the periods of appearing disconnected increased, and on some occasions Gary would breathe noisily, as if he was asleep and snoring.

Suspecting that Gary's behaviour was neurological rather than behavioural, the nurses took Gary to his GP and, after tests and hospital examination a diagnosis of epilepsy was made. While this is not unusual in clients with a learning disability, the diagnosis of epilepsy confirmed that Gary had altered neurological functioning, possibly affecting his general behaviour. Commencing with medication, Gary's nurses then began to re-plan his care, with renewed emphasis on safeguarding his physical and emotional wellbeing.

People with a learning disability have a brain disorder that variously affects the person's ability to deal with information. There can be difficulties in receiving and/or processing and/or transmitting processes in the brain, often first noticed when the person experiences problems with their speed of learning. People who have a learning disability typically have difficulty performing skills or tasks that people without a learning disability find straightforward to learn, for example dressing, finding their way around the locality, cleaning their teeth, opening a packet.

A common misconception is that having a learning disability means that the person is of lower intelligence. This is not correct, although recognising what might be called 'intelligent behaviours' may be more difficult than in most people.

There are many different types of learning disability, all caused by impaired or disrupted development of the brain. As our brains are almost fully formed before we are born it follows that most learning disabilities arise in the foetus, during birth or from serious illness in the early childhood years. Unlike many areas of health care, where the problem or need is often for a relatively short part of life, learning disability is a 'whole life' challenge which will have a significant impact on the way the person lives their life and gains independence.

For many people it is not possible to be certain of the cause(s) of their learning disability, but the following causes can sometimes be determined.

Environmental causes

■ **The developing foetus.** Formation of the central nervous system (brain and spinal cord) starts very early, at a stage when the mother may not be aware that she is pregnant. If the mother experiences illness or trauma or is exposed to harmful situations or substances, there can be impairment of brain development in the foetus.

■ **Hypoxia in childbirth.** If the baby is starved of oxygen at the time of birth, for example if the mother becomes ill, the brain can be damaged, causing temporary ill health or often permanent damage with subsequent learning disability.

■ **Early childhood illness or trauma.** Some serious injuries or illnesses in the first few years of life can damage the brain, either directly (e.g.

tumours, meningitis), or indirectly (e.g. severe respiratory or cardiac problems, which can result in insufficient oxygen reaching the brain).

Genetic causes

Genetic disorders are passed to the child from a parent. There are many rare and complex disorders: two common causes of learning disability are Down's syndrome – everyone who has this has a learning disability – and Fragile X syndrome – many but not all people who have this have a learning disability. Such syndromes are not learning disabilities in themselves.

Early in the pregnancy there can also be genetic mutation in the developing infant.

Living with a learning disability

We now know that human learning starts well before we are born. We can be certain of this because in addition to basic reflex actions such as sucking, healthy newborn babies have a range of highly developed behaviours through which they can interact with their environment. In a newborn infant we can see the baby discriminate between smells, sounds and visual stimuli and we see the capability to learn immediately present, for example, imitating facial expressions, responding to repeated tones or voices. Understanding a little about the significance of learning in the foetus and newborn child helps us appreciate the impact that disabled learning can have on a person – learning is fundamental to our development, as almost all of our behaviours are learned.

The overall incidence of learning disability, at least in most developed countries, is about 2% of the population – just over one million people in the UK. Of course, as in physical health impairment, there is a diverse range of disability level, with loose descriptions of mild, moderate, severe and profound learning disability being widely used. Approximately 0.3% of the whole population are regarded as having a severe or profound learning disability – or just over 200,000 people in the UK. In the future it is likely that there will be more people with a learning disability. This is because:

■ there are increasing survival rates among infants and children with severe and profound learning disability

■ increased survival rates of very premature or ill infants

Marcus, now 19, has a series of profound and complex learning disabilities complicated by physical health needs including diabetes, dysphagia, arthritis and osteoporosis.

case STUDY

Marcus has never been able to stand unaided or to walk. He needs 24/7 personal care, some of which, for example hoisting in/out of a wheelchair/bed/lavatory, needs two staff members.

For some people Marcus might appear to have a limited quality of life yet nothing could be further from the truth! When Marcus feels well he thoroughly enjoys his music (pop classics), dancing (in a wheelchair!), parties and meeting up with his family. Good though this is, in reality there are many days when Marcus does not feel well enough to enjoy life and difficulty with communication means it is not easy for his nurses to ascertain why he is less responsive than on 'good days'. The diabetes too makes life difficult, with Marcus's blood glucose levels being unstable, needing finger-prick blood tests and insulin injections three times a day.

Marcus lives in a community residence adapted for his needs; four other young clients with learning disabilities, each of whom has additional health needs, share the house. With their extended and complex needs Marcus and his house friends have their care directed by a trained learning disability nurse on a full-time basis, supported by a team of health care assistants. Each has an individual health needs assessment and plan, which is reviewed daily.

- adults with a learning disability are living longer
- in the UK at least, an increasing proportion of the population is from South Asian ethnic families, amongst whom rates of learning disability are higher.

One issue that is clear is that people with a learning disability do not have the same control over their own lives as other people in the community: they regularly face challenges and prejudice, and many, probably most, people with a learning disability are treated as 'different'.

Some of the common issues of learning disability that can impact on daily life are listed below.

- Around 80% of children with a learning disability are bullied.

- Someone with a learning disability is between six and eight times more likely to die before they are 50 years old, compared with people without a learning disability.

- Less than 30% of adults of working age with a learning disability are in any form of employment; most who do work do so part time for very low pay.

- Families where a child has a learning disability are more likely to live in poverty than other families.

- People with a learning disability have less opportunity to live independently and make choices – at least half of all adults who have a learning disability live in the family (their parental) home.

- In the UK around 30,000 adults with a learning disability live with parents who are over 70 years old, many of whom struggle with the caring roles they wish to fulfil but now find challenging.

- Up to 30% of people with a learning disability also have problems with their mental health, for example anxiety/neuroses or depression.

There is also a greater risk of associated physical ill health for people with a learning disability:

- diabetes is common

- epilepsy is 25% more common than in people without learning disabilities

- impaired vision is 50% more common

- respiratory infections, often severe, are much more common.

As we saw with Gary earlier in this chapter, some people with learning disabilities can also experience challenging behaviour which interferes with the physical safety of the person or other people. Examples include behaviours which are verbally or physically aggressive, self-harm or intensely repetitive actions. The reasons for challenging behaviours are often unknown but can include associated mental ill health, medication or pain, or be a learned way of attracting attention. What is challenging behaviour to one person may be seen differently by others, yet it is always distressing for the individual, families and carers.

Learning disability is not …

Autism or an **autistic spectrum disorder** affects about half a million people in the UK; it is a condition affecting the way people communicate with other people and relate to their environment. People have autism throughout life and comprehend the world as a place without order; behaviourally they have difficulty in forming relationships and struggle to understand and express themselves to others. Autism is not a learning disability although approximately 50% of people with autism are thought to have a learning disability. People with autism alone are supported by educational psychologists, GPs and often by local and national charitable advisers.

Asperger's syndrome is a form of autism in which sufferers find social gatherings especially problematic. Sufferers have difficulties with understanding emotional expression and communication, particularly when trying to interpret the way other people express themselves visually or with their tone of voice. People with Asperger's have fewer problems expressing themselves and are less likely to have a learning disability than people who have autism. People with Asperger's syndrome find a regular routine helpful and reassuring, often becoming distressed if routines are disrupted.

Cerebral palsy is not a learning disability, but a high proportion of people with cerebral palsy also have a learning disability. It is a structural problem of the neurological system, caused by a part of the brain not developing properly before birth or during infancy. The impact of cerebral palsy can be very varied, from negligible to significant impairment of speech, mobility and movement.

Dyslexia is a specific learning difficulty (not a learning disability) that mainly affects the acquisition, development and use of language skills and literacy. People with **dyscalculia** have difficulty with acquiring number skills, number concepts and using numbers in arithmetic – it might be thought of as 'dyslexia with numbers'. Severe dyslexia and/or dyscalculia can have a major impact on daily life, learning and employment; however, they are specific learning difficulties rather than learning disabilities. People with significant dyslexia or dyscalculia are usually assisted and supported by education staff, for example teachers. The prevalence of dyslexia and dyscalculia is not fully understood – estimates for the UK range from 2% to 15% and 1% to 7% respectively, depending on the distinction between mild and severe cases.

ROLE OF THE LEARNING DISABILITY NURSE

Learning disability nurses help their patients – usually referred to as 'clients' – to live their lives as independently as possible and to enjoy life as much as possible. Clients can be of any age – child to adult – but as life expectancy of people with a learning disability increases, there is a steady rise in the age profile of those supported.

Supporting the wellbeing and promoting the social inclusion of people with a learning disability is achieved by: helping individuals to maintain or improve their physical health; helping them maintain mental wellbeing; breaking down barriers; and engaging in tailored learning strategies to enhance independence. Progress may be in very small steps: for example, independence in oral/dental hygiene will not only benefit personal health but also reduce carer intervention; similarly, learning and carrying out safe practice to get to a shop or a friend's house independently has a positive impact both on the individual (giving them greater freedom) and family or carers (in terms of time and cost).

All nurses work both independently and as part of a team, with learning disability nurses distinctively working as key practitioners with interdisciplinary and multi-agency teams. Previously in the UK, most clients with a learning disability were cared for through NHS services, most frequently in institutions, often 'mental handicap hospitals', some distance from towns, families and friends. This system was, correctly, criticised for being impersonal, limiting choice and opportunities for clients to have time with family/education/employment, and restricting social activities. Since the 1980s there has been progress in introducing and delivering community care policy, which has changed the whole pattern of care for people with a learning disability and encouraged the delivery of support and care for people in their own homes wherever possible. In addition to the obvious benefits in terms of individual rights, choices and freedoms, community care has also been demonstrated to be less expensive and standards of care higher. In terms of actually ensuring that care works, significant changes to practices have led to most UK clients receiving care from a partnership of providers, including the NHS, social care agencies such as local authorities/social services, housing associations, education centres and, significantly, charities such as Mencap.

Lesley, 28, has just started her final year of training.

I'm in my final year of a learning disability nursing course. Before I started my training I had worked with adults who had learning disabilities for nearly 10 years. I found, initially to my own surprise, that I really enjoyed working with the clients, most of whom were a lot older than I was. One of things I found most rewarding, at least with my clients, was that they were just such lovely people who really appreciated me being there as a friend as well as a helper (I was there as a part-time health care assistant (HCA) while my children were growing up). Studying to be a qualified nurse has opened my eyes so much to all the research and theory of nursing that I am now putting into practice – I wish I had known all this when I was an HCA.

One of the best bits of the course has been the range of placements, which has hugely expanded my repertoire of skills and knowledge. My experiences have included working with children who have a learning disability; in a mental health acute admissions unit; in a young offenders institution – they had a secure unit for clients with learning disability who had committed serious crime; in a hospice; in a supported employment service for adults with a learning disability; and in community homes, one of which was run by a charity, the other by the NHS. When I qualify next year, I hope to get a job that will enable me to co-ordinate care services between the different providers as I believe this is vital to help drive up standards of care for our clients.

In the team of professional providers for people with a learning disability, nurses are frequently the lead practitioner. Typical day-to-day roles include:

- collaborating with fellow professionals to assess clients and develop personalised plans of care

- teaching clients strategies to help them live more independently; this might range from cleaning teeth or dressing to cooking or making journeys

- encouraging and facilitating clients to engage in education, employment, family life, parenting

- acting as an advocate for the client

- supporting physical and mental wellbeing, for example involving healthy eating, communication, de-escalating stressful/anxious situations

- supporting the families of clients and/or their carers, for example by facilitating respite care, teaching new ways of caring, listening.

Learning disability nurses often work with clients in either their family home or supported accommodation, for example a house which has been adapted to become the home of perhaps four clients. Learning disability nurses also work with clients who have more intensive or extended needs, perhaps in a hospital setting – for clients with complex needs, such as challenging behaviour, or who have physical ill health – in order to support clients for whom effective communication may not be possible.

Places of employment for learning disability nurses include:

- residential settings, including local homes in the community – these services may be managed by the NHS or independent providers or charities
- prisons/custody centres/young offender institutions
- acute hospitals, supporting clients with a learning disability
- mental health services, especially supporting clients with challenging behaviour
- schools or special schools, often with residential provision
- adult education settings
- supported employment services
- forensic/secure services for adults or children
- the independent sector
- nursing homes
- day centres, e.g. those managed by social services
- local authorities/housing providers
- advocacy services
- NHS Direct.

In settings such as this, learning disability nurses will work closely with:

- doctors
- health visitors
- client advocates
- mental health nurses
- dentists
- dietitians
- housing advisers
- benefits advisers
- physiotherapists and/or fitness staff

- voluntary agencies
- speech and language therapists
- occupational therapists
- family members
- health care assistants
- social workers
- teachers
- employers
- court services
- psychologists.

Zakariya, 32, is an experienced learning disability nurse.

I knew that I wanted to care for other people since I was 14, after I helped my parents take a cousin with Downs syndrome on holiday. After a few days I had begun to work out how my cousin communicated his needs – a mix of words and pointing – and I really enjoyed our time together; we have spent a lot of time together since then!

I began my training as a learning disability nurse in 1999, initially thinking that all the clients would be like my cousin. Of course I was wrong, and what I particularly liked was the concept of using evidence from past experiences or research to inform new practice, in other words learning through professional reflection to initiate evidence-based practice. Over my training I spent one extended placement working with clients who had complex needs, some of whom were or had been alcohol or drug dependent; some of these clients had been in prison for committing a range of offences, although I was clear in my own mind that for at least some of them, the need was for professional care, not criminal punishment. Once qualified, I worked in several different roles, giving me experience with a wide range of clients; I also worked as a volunteer with a national charity concerned with the welfare of prisoners – of course I remained passionately interested in the needs of people with a learning disability who were held in custody.

Now, I am fortunate in having a role as project manager for a large charity, my job being to resettle people who have a learning disability from custody settings to more permanent residential care in local communities. I work closely with prisons and young offenders units, the police, local communities, social workers, voluntary organisations, social services, housing providers, the probation service … and, of course, learning disability nurses working in the community. My aim is to help people with often complex learning disabilities live fulfilled and valued lives within their local community.

LEARNING DISABILITY NURSING: THE COURSE

University education is half of the course leading to registration as a learning disability nurse, and includes areas of study such as:

- professional and ethical practices

- ethical and legal responsibilities

- communication strategies

- advocacy for clients and their families

- safeguarding clients, including safe administration of medication

- working to support individual rights and anti-discrimination

- political, economic and societal context of care

- delivering care to clients of all ages and in all settings through:

  - assessment strategies and practices

  - using evidence to support practice

  - health promotion

☐ life and social sciences

☐ developing clinical care skills

■ managing and leading care through:

☐ co-ordinating care pathways on an interprofessional basis

☐ advising and educating clients and other professionals

☐ developing practices in response to updated research and community needs

☐ innovative and challenging care in response to clients' and families' needs.

The other half of the course is placement, with a range of opportunities provided for you to gain insight into and experience of the range of clients receiving learning disability nursing care in the local area. Experiences will normally include a wide range of ages, dependences and behaviours, including working with people who exhibit challenging behaviour; there is often a period of 'extended client attachment' during which, while supervised, you take increasing responsibility for a client over a period of many months. Students will work with their clients in NHS, local authority, independent (private) and charitable settings – in fact anywhere clients are cared for and supported professionally. Students can expect to be supervised and mentored by both experienced learning disability nurses and other registered and relevant professionals.

While retaining their independence as registered nurses and accountability for their practice, learning disability nurses frequently share responsibility for their clients with an extended multidisciplinary team. These interprofessional teams often share a single client assessment – health, mental, social and other needs – planning and delivering care or services together. This requires high standards of communication and flexible working, yet gives opportunity for a much more holistic and cost-effective plan of care that avoids duplication. Promoting and delivering such cohesive care also helps avoid gaps and maintains standards in care provision.

ESSENTIAL SKILLS

Learning disability nurses engage with and care for an exceptional group of individuals across the whole age spectrum. An effective learning disability nurse often exhibits qualities from all the other areas of nursing and many other health professions. The qualities needed are distinctive, perhaps exemplified by the need for patience, as the rewards from interventions and care are often delayed. Universities, health and social care providers work together to select for and deliver learning disability nurse training and prepare for future employment. Some useful core skills and attributes are:

- excellent and sensitive verbal and non-verbal communication skills with all ages and all groups in society

- the ability to learn alternative means of communication

- a genuine interest in all people – disabled and non-disabled

- a caring and affable personality

- emotional resilience

- patience and determination

- reliable and consistent listening

- excellent and dependable communication skills with staff colleagues from many professions, disciplines and sectors

- the ability to engage sensitively with clients of all backgrounds, cultures and beliefs and to learn (assess) from this

- recognition of confidentiality of information, including to/from/ between family members

- the potential to learn how to respond to distressed clients

- confidence in talking with people who cannot communicate or respond easily

- the ability to use intuition, recognising one's own boundaries and limitations

- as training progresses, the ability to learn how to and then to make decisions

- the potential to cope with difficult or distressing ethical situations

- the ability to observe details, especially even minor changes from the 'norm'

- consistency and reliability; a professional approach
- personal integrity.

WHY LEARNING DISABILITY NURSING?

The purpose of this chapter has been to help you explore what learning disability nursing is, and what it is not. For many practitioners it is the opportunity for extended caring relationships with clients that draws them to this area of nursing care, together with the prospect of being a lead professional among so many other team members. Learning disability nurses are special – caring, compassionate, strong in their commitment to evidence-based practice, and patient, with a determination to progress their client's independence.

Chapter Seven
MIDWIFERY

WHAT IS MIDWIFERY?

To many people, perhaps the majority, the role of a midwife is to deliver babies. Of course, midwives are certainly key practitioners in assisting women to deliver their babies, yet important though this is, the role extends professional care and support of women to both before and after a birth. In fact, the term 'midwife' is derived from an Old English word meaning 'with woman'.

Birth rates tend to follow trends over a number of years; at the time of preparing this book rates have been slowly increasing for several years to over 750,000 births annually in the UK and over 70,000 in Ireland. To set the context of midwifery practice, a brief overview of the nature of midwifery care is helpful. Midwives' roles include:

- care and advice during pregnancy
- preparation of mother and perhaps others for parenthood
- responsibility for managing labour and childbirth
- postpartum (post-birth) care of the mother
- postnatal (post-birth) care of the infant
- promotion of normal birth
- assessment of mother and baby, e.g. identification of any complications
- liaising with other health care professionals

■ family planning

■ assistive reproduction

■ education for parent(s), family and community

■ support/advice/counselling for women to achieve or maintain good sexual and reproductive health.

Historically, supporting the process of birth was the job of the local 'handywoman' or attendant, a practice still commonplace in developing countries. Such women frequently have no formal training but have often had several children themselves and have experience of assisting birthing women. In the UK, the Midwives' Act in 1902 formalised the training of midwives, essential to be permitted to practise; nowadays it is the NMC that regulates the training that must be undertaken, monitoring and assessing both the quality and standards of training and providing a code of professional conduct to which midwives must adhere.

For most women, pregnancy is normal and birth is straightforward – this should be expected since, of course, pregnancy and childbirth are essentially healthy processes. This and other factors make midwifery a distinctly different profession from all areas of nursing, each of which supports people whose health is compromised or disrupted.

Midwives identify that their 'client group' has changed in the past few decades, in particular with a stretching of the age profile. In the UK, the current youngest mother was just 11 years old when she gave birth, the oldest 66 years old. While these are certainly the exception, Britain has a consistently very high teenage pregnancy and birth rate and simultaneously, a steady trend of older mothers.

Other changes to the client groups midwives work with include:

■ homeless women

■ victims of domestic violence, asylum seekers

■ women who have a learning disability or mental health need

■ drug misusers

■ mothers who are HIV- or hepatitis-positive

■ women who have limited or no use of the English language.

Loretta, 54, is a community midwife.

case STUDY

I qualified in 1978 – I must be nearly the oldest midwife around! Having worked on a variety of maternity wards I then began to take a keen interest in the community. I think this was the impact of having my own three children interfacing with other mums at school, and just generally growing up! I work with a colleague out of a GP surgery covering a small town. After I have initially booked a mother in, I then maintain contact with antenatal visits (they come to me) and my colleague and I are both on call for them when they go into labour. In addition to the assessment of mothers and their unborn babies I also run regular antenatal classes, an aqua-natal class [water-based exercise during and after pregnancy] at the local leisure centre and have just completed a course so I can offer baby massage classes.

One thing I have as a community midwife, but didn't have in the hospital, is time to prioritise personal or individual support. I think this is really important as for most women, pregnancy is the first time they have had concentrated input from a health professional. I am passionate about making use of my skills and opportunities to offer (and that's all it can ever be) support for my mothers to eat more healthily, consider their non-pregnant weight, stop smoking and avoid excessive alcohol. I also come across a number whose lifestyle seems incompatible with a long and healthy life.

I get a huge amount of satisfaction from midwifery – 'my mums' are really special!

Midwives within the health care system

For many women, midwives are the only health care professionals involved during pregnancy. However, if an aspect of the woman's pregnancy appears to fall outside the normal expectations, the midwife 'escalates', referring her to a colleague appropriate to the need, for example an obstetrician or a physiotherapist. After delivery of the infant, the midwife will continue to be involved in monitoring and assessing the health of both mother and baby, normally for 28 days.

In the UK, the NHS is by far the largest employer of midwives – around 22,000 in total. However, there are many other employment opportunities for midwives to consider.

- **Antenatal and postnatal wards.** Most NHS maternity hospitals have in-patient ward areas supporting women with antenatal (pre-birth) and postnatal (post-birth) care. Antenatal care may involve women experiencing complications such as pre-eclampsia, a condition potentially harmful (even fatal) to both mother and baby. Postnatal care includes care of women (and their babies) where birth has been difficult or traumatic, for example where surgical repair or caesarean section has been necessary.

- **Labour wards.** All NHS hospital maternity units have a labour ward, an emergency admission unit for pregnant women mainly focused on the labour and delivery area. Labour wards may be led by an obstetrician (a medical consultant specialising in pregnancy), a family doctor/GP, a midwife or a combination of all these. Appropriate specialist services are available, for example epidural anaesthesia, birth pool, close links to operating theatres and high dependency unit (HDU) to support women with severe complications of pregnancy.

- **Foetal care centres.** Specialist foetal care centres may be provided by NHS or independent (private) hospitals. They support mothers/parents where a baby may have been identified as having an antenatal problem, and offer dedicated care.

- **Community midwives.** Community midwives offer antenatal and postnatal care for women in their own homes; home births are also attended, although these remain relatively uncommon in the UK. In team midwifery a mother is supported by a number of midwives who work in both community and hospital; one benefit is that the mother builds a professional relationship with a number of midwives during the antenatal period. Community midwives are most commonly employed by the NHS, although a smaller number work independently.

- **Birth centres** are midwife-led units (either NHS or private). They can be either based in a hospital or separate from it. Birth centres are sometimes described as a halfway house between home and hospital births, offering a relaxed atmosphere in a well-equipped and midwife-staffed environment. Facilities are likely to include low-tech birthing rooms, a birth pool, massage and a 'menu' of analgesia (pain relief).

- **Independent midwifery.** Independent midwifery offers more autonomy for the midwife, who can choose to take on as many or as few mothers as she/he wants and can professionally care for. Most care, including deliveries, takes place in the mother's own home. The job offers much satisfaction, but it does mean being 'on call' for 'your' mothers 24/7.

- **Military.** The armed forces employ a small number of midwives, primarily to support the civilian wives and partners of serving personnel.

- **Fertility/assisted conception** services are provided by both the state and independent health providers. Some services that are typically available are in vitro fertilisation, hormone therapy and frozen embryos (e.g. associated with cancer treatment). The role of the midwife, working in the context of complex moral and ethical considerations, includes pre-conception advice to prospective parents, for example on nutrition, health lifestyle or behaviours.

- **Health visiting.** Midwives (or nurses) may train as health visitors, providing they have at least one year's experience. Health visitor training is usually a pathway offered as part of a university's specialist community nursing programme, often at master's degree level.

- **Other roles.** Other opportunities for midwives include working as a supervisor of midwives, lecturer, practice development manager, service manager, Sure Start midwife. For more information on these roles, see Chapter 8.

Justin is delivered at home.

First I asked the hospital midwife, then my GP, then the obstetrician – they were all emphatically against home delivery for a first child. There was a range of excuses, mostly because they said I was too big. I agree that I am slightly obese but looking through the information on the internet I could find nothing to indicate that a slightly obese mum was high risk for home delivery. My problem with hospitals is that they frighten me. They are all so big and noisy and you end up in a 'bedroom' with lots of strangers – they aren't strange people – just not the people you would choose to share a hotel room with! I guess I'm also a bit frightened because my sister was very ill when I was young and she later died at the same hospital where my maternity unit is.

Having been emphatic that I wasn't going to deliver in hospital, I was referred to a birthing centre about 15 miles from home. I had a good look round and as the leaflet said, it was a bit like home – a home with hospital beds! To be perfectly honest it wasn't too bad but I had started out by insisting on a home delivery and the very friendly midwife who showed me round was very sympathetic. She explained that there were some risks to a home delivery, for example if the baby got stuck or if I lost too much blood – I would then need an ambulance and there would be no guarantee that baby or I would be okay. I went back to see the birthing centre midwife again and she agreed that the team of midwives would support me to deliver at home – I whooped so loudly!

After a number of antenatal visits when the midwife talked my partner and me through the preparations needed at home, I was ready! At 10.00 p.m. my waters broke – I cried – and left partner to clear up! We phoned the midwife and she came out. After examining me, checking my blood pressure and baby's heart rate she said to go to bed, as tomorrow might be a long day. The next morning I began having painful cramping-type sensations in my abdomen and thighs, my midwife reappeared, performed an internal examination, pronounced that I was four centimetres dilated and now in labour. She predicted that I would be a mum by tea time.

After the midwife had gone I had breakfast, phoned my own mother and had a bath to try to relax. I had always thought that the baby would drown, but for me it was very relaxing despite the contractions. By 11.00 a.m. the contractions were very regular and long, they were also very painful as the relaxation of the bath seemed to have worn off very quickly. The midwife reappeared with a supply of Entonox gas [analgesia], which certainly helped. The next hour or so is just a little hazy but … just after midday Justin arrived, all 8lb 5oz of him – very healthy and with a healthy, satisfied but tired mum!

WHAT DO MIDWIVES DO?

The exact role of a midwife will normally vary from day to day and is very variable depending on the setting being worked in. Bearing this in mind, the following gives a brief overview.

- Assessing the baby's heartbeat using a stethoscope or electronic foetal monitor. This may be done regularly or continuously (in labour) and periodically in the antenatal period.

- Vaginal examination to see if or how far the mother's cervix has dilated: this gives a good indication of progression in labour.

- Supporting women with increasing ethnic diversity, including asylum seekers and migrant families who have limited use of English.

- Checking the mother's blood pressure: this is done regularly during labour and periodically in the antenatal period.

- Assessing the stage of labour.

- Confirming pregnancy, then monitoring and examining women during pregnancy.

- Assessing the mother, then developing, delivering and evaluating individual programmes of care.

- Screening tests in the hospital, community and the home; includes blood tests.

- Identifying higher-risk pregnancies and making referrals to doctors and other members of the multidisciplinary team.

- Facilitating or providing parenting and health education for the mother, her partner/husband and perhaps other family members.

- Encouraging the partner/husband/birthing friend to support the mother during labour.

- Providing counselling and advice following events such as miscarriage, termination of pregnancy, stillbirth, birth abnormality and neonatal death.

- Supervising and assisting mothers in labour and monitoring the condition of the foetus.

- Prescribing and administering medications, especially analgesics.

- Giving advice on the daily care of the infant, including promotion of breast feeding, and bathing.

- Participating in the training and supervision of junior colleagues.

- Advising on nutrition and fluid intake.

- Episiotomy (cutting the perineal skin to prevent tearing); later suturing (stitching) and administering local anaesthesia.

- Suturing tears in the perineum.

- Supporting women to choose and use different positions during labour.

MIDWIFERY: THE COURSE

There are currently two ways of training to become a midwife:

1 A direct-entry full-time course offered by a university in collaboration with its NHS partners. Once completed this option will give you two 'awards' – an academic award from the university (usually a

bachelor's degree) and the opportunity to register as a midwife with the NMC. There is no nursing involved. Direct-entry courses are already the most common preparation, a trend likely to continue. The course is 50% supervised practice and 50% academic study. Competition for places is intense.

2   Midwifery short programme – for qualified and registered nurses (usually adult nurses) wishing to train as midwives. The course lasts a minimum of 18 months, and involves a similar amount of supervised practice as in the three-year course. There is considerable competition for places; this programme currently has very restricted availability in the UK.

When choosing the undergraduate degree route, university education is half of the course leading to registration as a midwife, and it includes areas of study such as:

- professional and ethical practices

- ethical and legal responsibilities

- communication strategies, including where English is not spoken

- advocacy for mothers of all cultures/ethnicities

- safeguarding, including safe administration of medication

- a woman-centred approach

- political, economic and societal context of maternal care

- delivering equitable care to women through:

  - □ normal antenatal, intrapartum (during childbirth) and postnatal care

  - □ complex antenatal, intrapartum and postnatal care

  - □ promoting positive health messages to women and families (e.g. giving up smoking)

  - □ care of the healthy and compromised neonate

- life and social sciences

- pharmacology

- managing and leading care through:

  ☐ autonomous midwifery practice

  ☐ advising and educating clients, families and other professionals

  ☐ decision making and clinical maternal health leadership

  ☐ identifying, using and extending the evidence base for maternal health care

  ☐ innovative and challenging care in response to the needs of women.

The other half of a midwifery course is placement, with a range of opportunities designed to help you gain insight into and experience the depth and breadth of maternal health and to achieve the necessary and statutory experiences. As your course develops, and remaining fully supervised, you will take increasing responsibility for your practice, including a number of normal and complex births as well as antenatal and postnatal assessments and associated care. Placements may include periods of being 'on call'. Experience will be gained in both community and maternity hospital settings. It is common to have a supervised caseload of women where you take increasingly independent responsibility for mothers. Students will normally be supervised and mentored by experienced midwives.

Samantha, aged 26, is a labour ward midwife.

In 2004 I went straight to university from college, after gaining three B grades for my A levels – I was very pleased with my achievements then but better was to come! From a young age – about 12 – I had liked the idea of new life, of the amazing processes women went through to deliver their babies successfully. I think part of the initial learning and motivation was from a documentary series on television – a fly on the wall 'real life' insight – in which I had been particularly grabbed by the amount of preparation before delivery – I had naively thought women just turned up to deliver the baby! I also liked the idea that in midwifery, the women or 'clients' were not ill – they had need for support but rarely were they really unwell.

Having achieved my A levels I decided to move away from home, only about 50 miles away, but it meant my mum couldn't just pop round, although I could go home if I needed to. My course was a BSc in Midwifery. There were 22 other girls, mostly my age, plus one man. We had six weeks of introductory lectures; I thought at the time that they were dull and uninteresting – lots of anatomy and physiology – yet as soon as we got into practice I realised the importance of knowing what goes where and how the different body systems affect the wellbeing of the mother. My first placement was six weeks on an antenatal ward – this felt really scary, even though we didn't have the urgency of deliveries happening all around us.

When I went into the labour ward for the first time I have to confess that I cried at my first birth; funnily enough, I still cry now at most births I attend as the emotions run so high. Qualifying in 2007, I find my job now to be stressful but manageable – there are days when we barely have enough beds and staff sickness makes delivering high-quality care difficult – but this is my job, always ensuring that delivered care is to a really high standard.

ESSENTIAL SKILLS

When you apply for midwifery training at university the selection process is always led by registered midwives from the university and their midwife colleagues from practice. With entry highly competitive at most good universities, selectors are looking for the range of skills that will enable the candidate to engage with a three-year degree programme and to be a high-quality future midwife. Wherever possible, some evidence of exploring these skills in practice – relevant voluntary work for example – is particularly valued. To support preparation, it is useful to begin to highlight your own personal qualities, perhaps in a journal or diary, noting how you have gained or used each talent or ability. The following are recognised as essential attributes of a midwife:

- excellent and sensitive verbal and non-verbal communication skills with all ages and all groups in society

- being prepared to care for all women and their families irrespective of class, ethnicity, age, sexuality or beliefs

- a genuine desire to be involved in personal care without regard for prejudice or objection to unpleasant circumstance

- the ability to remain calm and objective in an emergency situation

- a caring and affable personality

- the ability to work well independently and as part of a team

- excellent and dependable communication skills with staff colleagues of many professions, disciplines and sectors

- recognition of the importance of confidentiality of information, including to/from/between family members

- the potential to learn how to break bad news

- confidence in talking with adults, including people you don't know

- the ability to use intuition, recognising boundaries and limitations

- as training progresses, the ability to learn how to make decisions

- the ability to observe detail, especially even minor changes from the 'norm'

- consistency and reliability

- a professional approach

- personal integrity

- physical and emotional stamina.

WORKING INTERPROFESSIONALLY

Midwives are registered and accountable practitioners, taking personal responsibility for their professional practice and often working autonomously. Whether working independently or in a team, and regardless of where they are working, almost all midwives work as part of an interprofessional or multidisciplinary team. Interprofessional learning is a strong component of all good midwifery training courses.

For midwives the interprofessional team will be likely to include obstetricians, physiotherapists, social workers, doctors/surgeons, neonatologists, housing advisers, diabetes staff, benefits advisers, medical scientists, dietitians, education providers, ultrasound technicians and all types of nurse.

WHY MIDWIFERY?

We have learned that midwives have a range of roles and responsibilities, almost entirely focused on the care of the mother, and it is worth reaffirming that it is a misconception that midwives work primarily with babies! With the intensity of competition for training places it is vital to prepare yourself and your application carefully, gaining as much relevant experience as possible before submitting a meticulously prepared application. Getting it right opens up one of the most rewarding professions on earth!

Chapter Eight
RELATED CAREER ROLES IN NURSING AND MIDWIFERY

THE ARMED FORCES

The armed forces of many countries, including the UK, are large-scale employers of nurses, especially those trained in adult or mental health nursing. A common misconception is that nursing in the military is all about front-line duties, but this is only one of the many locations of deployment.

Adult nurses working in the military may find themselves working in any of a particularly broad range of locations, working autonomously or with medical teams to provide specialist nursing support in environments that may be unpredictable. The range of responsibilities and opportunities is not dissimilar to that found in civilian employment, but experiences can sometimes be intense and time-pressured, as patient assessment and management decisions may need to be made rapidly. Particularly useful areas of practice include:

- trauma/accident and emergency/triage

- operating theatres, including surgical assisting, recovery and anaesthetics

- intensive and critical care

- all surgical settings, especially orthopaedics

- all neurological specialities

- in-flight emergency repatriation

- acute medicine

- 'community' work with members of the armed forces and their families

- health screening and occupational health

- tropical diseases within military and local civilian communities.

Mental health nurses working in the armed forces manage a caseload of personnel with diverse mental health care needs. This may be on operational duties, linked with peacekeeping roles or in teams supporting the armed forces community – both military and civilian.

An extensive set of skills and relevant knowledge is needed as situations encountered can be challenging and change rapidly. Nurses work with military and civilian colleagues in the home country and on postings abroad. Mental health nursing in the military can be an excellent place to be supported in your professional development, and for those who demonstrate leadership qualities, officer commissions are available. Nurses are likely to encounter clients with a similar range of mental health disorders as found in civilians, but these are often exacerbated by traumatic or upsetting experiences, especially among those in front-line combatant roles. Problems such as post-traumatic stress disorder may be encountered more frequently.

Both adult and mental health nurses in the armed forces may work in a land-based hospital or clinic in their home country, on ships, in military bases in the home country or overseas, in casualty settings or field hospitals near conflict areas or as part of a humanitarian aid team in areas affected by natural disaster. Support is often given to local communities if overseas and, of course, military personnel from both home countries and hostile combatants are cared for.

Although they are non-combatants, nurses are required to undertake basic military training skills and need to be physically fit. Many nurses in the armed forces are confident that not only do they use and extend the skills they would use in civilian nursing, but they also gain an extensive portfolio of unrivalled and unique military-specific nursing experiences.

Midwives are very rarely employed by the armed forces in the UK.

IN-FLIGHT NURSING: PATIENT REPATRIATION

This area of practice mostly employs adult-trained nurses, with occasional opportunities for those who are mental health nurses, children's nurses or midwives. In-flight nurses either work in the armed forces – Princess Mary's Royal Air Force Nursing Services in the UK – or, more commonly, for commercial services.

Nurses need to have gained experience in acute or critical care areas after qualifying and then undertake additional training in order to demonstrate that they can transfer their skills to in-flight settings. Commercial assistance companies provide repatriation and aeromedical services, typically for insurance companies, government departments and private individuals. Employment may be full time or freelance, with travel at short notice to absolutely anywhere. The patients being cared for are often critically ill, but stable, and nursing care may well be challenging and involve the use of life support equipment. Although involving extensive travel, the purpose of the journey is to work professionally – unfortunately, it is not a way of becoming a global tourist.

THE LEISURE INDUSTRY

Nurses – normally adult trained – are employed in a range of leisure industry settings including cruise ships and (both at home and overseas) in holiday parks, residential or activity centres, large leisure complexes and occasionally on expeditions.

For work in the cruise industry, for example, nurses need to consolidate their training – experience in acute medical and surgical wards, coronary care, A&E, intensive and similar critical care environments is particularly relevant; experience and qualification in advanced life support is often required. On large vessels you will be part of a very small team, perhaps two or three other nurses and a doctor. You will need to be able to think intuitively and make professional, independent decisions rapidly. Voyages and periods of work can be extended – perhaps for several months – before generous home leave; return flights are provided and salaries can be higher than on land with the additional benefits of full accommodation, food and your own leisure opportunities.

NURSING HOMES

Nursing homes (whether run privately or by the NHS, local authorities or charitable groups) are large-scale employers of both adult and mental health nurses. Nurses need to have an aptitude for delivering high-quality and often complex care to clients for whom the nursing home is their home – often permanently. Clients could be of any age and could have a diverse range of nursing care needs. They are often, through physical disability or illness, unable to care for themselves; and they might include older residents who may be physically frail and/or have dementia. Standards of care are very high, with nurses often gaining strong support from their employer to extend their training and undertake management and leadership roles.

NHS DIRECT (UK)

The NHS Direct service enables the public to obtain telephone health advice from registered nurses, who use a system of computer-based decision guidelines and algorithms to determine appropriate advice tailored to the needs of the enquirer. Callers present with an extremely broad range of enquiries: some can be resolved by simple self-care; others need urgent referral to paramedic or hospital services.

Opportunities in NHS Direct are open to all trained nurses and midwives; a range of expertise is needed. Especially useful – where possible – is experience in A&E or critical care. Basic computer competence is helpful and, of course, a high standard of telephone communication skills is essential. As the roles are office based, they are sometimes a particularly useful opportunity for nurses or midwives who are limited by a disability.

PRISONS AND CUSTODY CENTRES

Opportunities for nursing in prisons are open to nurses who are adult, mental health or learning disability trained. In the UK, most prison nurses are employed by the NHS, though some are employed by the prison service or by commercial prison providers.

The patients and clients prison nurses work with typically have reduced 'civilian' engagement with health professionals, creating many opportunities for nurses to make positive contributions to health. Nursing in prison is sometimes seen as a development of practice nursing, yet the environment and often the patients are much more challenging. Nurses will often be supporting inmates:

■ with learning disabilities

■ who are previous and ongoing substance misusers

■ with diverse mental health needs

■ who have communicable diseases, including sexually transmitted infections

■ who self-harm

■ in pregnancy

■ where there is recognised disordered eating

■ with any physical health need or long-term condition

■ in need of health promotion/health choice messages

■ from many cultural and language backgrounds.

Prison nursing posts can sometimes be available for newly qualified as well as experienced nurses. Training opportunities are often very good, with continuing professional development and some openings to advance management and leadership skills and qualifications.

In recent years nurses have become increasingly employed in police custody centres, especially in larger cities. Clients and responsibilities are similar to prison nursing but may also involve assessment and examination of minor injuries and those who are alcohol intoxicated, also of victims of sexual or other assaults.

OCCUPATIONAL HEALTH NURSING

Occupational health nurses contribute to the health and wellbeing of employees in the workplace; many are employed by large companies – industrial, office and retail. Some occupational health nurses work as self-employed consultants. Most occupational health nurses are adult, or occasionally mental health, trained. Occupational health nursing roles typically include:

- risk assessment of the workplace for potential health and safety problems

- developing and implementing health and safeguarding policies

- delivering health promotion activities that are directly or indirectly work related

- delivering a range of health and health and safety training programmes

- contributing to accident follow-up

- monitoring employees whose jobs involve exposure to hazardous materials

- supporting employees to return to work after periods of ill health

- advising on workplace disability

- advising on overseas travel/providing vaccinations

- health screening of new employees.

Specialist qualification in occupational health nursing practice is available to nurses working in this area.

AID/MISSION/OVERSEAS CHARITABLE ROLES

Opportunities are available to all registered nurses and midwives, especially those with some post-qualification experience. It is usual for postings to be to some of the poorest and most impoverished parts of the world and to last for many months (aid/disaster relief) or several years (long-term development and missions). Except for some aid and disaster relief jobs with large international organisations (e.g. the United Nations, government agencies, International Red Cross), many nurses and midwives are employed by smaller charities on a voluntary basis or where pay is at the (very low) rate typical in the host country. It is often necessary to share or be sympathetic to the ethos of the organisation.

Almost any situation may be encountered, including very diverse and sometimes challenging nursing and maternal health needs. It is vital to be able to maintain professionalism but also think quickly, rationally and with cultural sensitivity. Resources are often extremely limited (e.g. intermittent electricity) and conditions and equipment basic, for example no blood transfusions or limited intravenous supplies, restricted or expensive medications, lack of clean/running water or difficulty in maintaining a clean environment. The range of needs encountered will include many of those experienced by patients in the UK/Europe and many more, including local/tropical disease and trauma/emergency situations that at home would be dealt with by a much more comprehensive team.

These are tremendously rewarding opportunities, literally life-changing for many people. There are occasionally opportunities for shorter-term roles.

TEACHING AND LECTURING

Nurse and midwife training is led by lecturers and clinical facilitators who are themselves experienced registered practitioners. It is helpful to have several years' experience in any relevant area of practice together with a higher-level academic qualification – at least an honours degree and preferably a master's-level qualification.

Employment is often by universities, where a mixed role of teaching and researching is common. Other opportunities are in further education and sixth-form colleges, supporting students undertaking health, social and child care courses. In addition, there are also many clinical education roles in the NHS, where it is possible to maintain regular clinical practice and support nursing or midwifery university students on placement experiences. Patterns of work are normally 'education hours' without weekend working.

SCHOOL NURSING

School nurses are children's nurses employed in any school setting, especially large independent/residential schools and schools supporting children with additional physical needs. They provide an essential link between health, school, home and the local community that helps safeguard the health and social wellbeing of children and young people. Support for the child's transition between child and adult services is also important.

A range of responsibilities can be expected, depending on the type of school, but may include:

- supporting children with complex health and medical needs (e.g. receiving kidney dialysis, neurological treatment, cerebral palsy)

- running clinics, both general and specific (e.g. for enuresis (bedwetting))

- immunisations and vaccinations

- annual health reviews, including, for example, monitoring body mass (weight)

- sexual health.

Conditions of employment can vary but can be better than national pay scales, for example accommodation and board may be provided and, depending on the school, holidays may be generous.

The NHS also employs school nurses on nationally agreed conditions. These are not residential posts but responsibilities are similar and involve extended links and referrals to and from other members of the community child health team.

Chapter Nine
TRAINING, SKILLS AND QUALIFICATIONS

In this chapter we will look at the qualifications and training required to become a nurse or midwife, at the skills you will need and how to go about getting some invaluable work experience.

It is important to remember that anyone hoping to enter nursing or midwifery will need to register with the NMC and must meet the entry requirements set by the organisation.

GENERAL SKILLS

What makes a good nurse or a midwife? Both careers are looking for people who have skills that will allow them to perform effectively in busy wards, clinics and community settings where no two days are ever the same. Everyone has skills that they acquire throughout their life. These skills will be shaped by the various facets of your life: your education, work, volunteering, travel and leisure activities. Skills acquired through being part of a sports team, community or voluntary group can sometimes be discounted, yet they can be just as important as those developed in the classroom, lecture theatre or workplace.

Anyone considering becoming a nurse needs to be:

- a good communicator who can listen, observe and give advice

- well organised and attentive to detail

- interested in caring for people

- calm, understanding and tactful when necessary

- a capable team worker who can work with a wide variety of health care colleagues and other professionals

- an effective problem solver who can evaluate situations and see a way forward

- resilient: some days will be challenging as well as rewarding.

If you are interested in training as a midwife you need to have all of the above skills and you also need to:

- have an interest in the process of pregnancy and birth, from scientific, psychological and social perspectives

- be a quick thinker who can react calmly to new situations

- be confident and mature, someone who will make women feel positive and in control

- be self-reliant and adaptable.

The NMC also expects applicants to have a suitable level of literacy, numeracy and good health. All applicants also have to be vetted by the Criminal Records Bureau.

All applicants whose first language is not English must obtain a minimum score of 7.0 in all sections of the International English Language Test.

WORK EXPERIENCE

Work experience can move you further forward from just having a career idea to actually gaining knowledge and understanding of the working environment that you hope to join. Work experience can be full time or part time, paid or unpaid, and it can be tailored around other aspects of your life such as education and family commitments. It is important to get relevant work experience before applying to train as a nurse or midwife – it will prove that you have an insight into health care and your chosen profession and it will also show that you are motivated and have gone beyond just thinking that you would like to train in either profession.

Many schools and colleges provide the opportunity for students to get involved in volunteering in health and social care organisations. Find out about what is available if you are still in education – getting involved in such schemes will certainly enhance your experience of caring for and supporting others. For many people, volunteering while at school or college is their first step towards understanding what the world of health care is really like and it can act as a catalyst for entering a career in many health and social care professions.

If you want to volunteer independently, many towns and cities in the UK have a volunteer bureau that can put you in touch with a relevant voluntary group to which you could offer your time. Volunteering with a local charity and providing support once a week for a year, for example, will give you a chance to really experience working in the care sector and will provide you with useful evidence for future applications. It will also give you the opportunity to experience the positive and negative aspects of care work, which will help you decide whether this type of employment is right for you.

Natalie Mihell, nursing applicant 2010.

I chose to apply to Southampton University to become a children's nurse as I always had the aspiration to work in a job in health care. At first I was unsure which course to take so I took some good advice, and undertook some voluntary work to see if I enjoyed working in a hospital and health care environment. At school I completed my Trident Work Experience at a nursery school, which I thoroughly enjoyed, therefore I decided to apply for voluntary work at my local hospital on the paediatric unit, due to my love of working with children. This really opened my eyes to the role of a children's nurse and what the job entails. I shadowed the nurses a lot and talked and played with the children to enable them to feel more comfortable and less vulnerable in their distressing times of need. I also became a helper at my local Rainbows, Brownies and Guides groups, which helped me gain confidence and develop the skills needed to work with children. Doing both of these things really helped confirm my decision to choose this branch of nursing at university.

Once I made this decision, I applied to four universities which offered this course. The four nearest to me were Southampton, Surrey, Bournemouth and Brighton, my first choice being Southampton. I wrote my personal statement and applied online through UCAS with the help of my college and then I just had to wait. I received letters from all of the universities with dates of interviews. The earliest date was Southampton, which I was so happy about. I wasn't sure if I would even get one interview, due to the competitiveness of the course and limited places. I was shortlisted from 600 applicants to one of 150 for interview.

I arrived at the interview dressed smartly and with some research material which we were allowed to bring for a group discussion we were going to have. First we had to complete short maths and English tests, which were fine. Next were our individual interviews, which I was completely terrified about, but the interviewers were really friendly, which put me at ease. It was more laid back than I thought it was going to be. They asked me why I chose this course and what I had done to make this decision, etc. I came out thinking it had gone quite well. We then had a group discussion where they were looking at our interpersonal skills and how we worked together in a team. Overall the interviewing process was quite nerve-racking but I just had to keep remembering to be myself and keep smiling! Nurses have to be smiley and friendly to make people feel comfortable. When I received the letter and notification through UCAS that they were offering me a place I was absolutely delighted and firmly accepted it straight away.

All in all I found the application process fairly easy, thanks to the help of college. The interview process was very quick and I found out I was successful within a week, so this made things much easier to handle. I am over the moon to have gained a place at my desired university, especially as the course is so competitive, and I cannot wait to start in September.

Paid employment in health care is another way of building up expertise. Local newspapers and recruitment agencies such as NHS Professionals and others advertise vacancies in hospitals, care homes, special needs schools and charities for care workers. Anyone wishing to become a midwife could also look at working in children's nurseries, children's centres and projects such as Sure Start. Building up relevant work experience will make you look credible when applying for a place on a higher education course at university. It will also give you first-hand experiences that you will be able to use in your university application and at interview.

Work shadowing

Work experience is important for entry to nursing and midwifery. Think hard about where you could gain relevant experience. If it is difficult to find experience in a very specific branch of nursing or midwifery, can you work shadow someone instead? Work shadowing involves spending time with someone in an occupation that interests you but where you might not be able to get actual experience. Anyone wishing to train as a midwife could spend a few hours with a community midwife – this is a great way to see what the role is really like. Use work shadowing as an opportunity to ask questions about the job that you are observing. Before meeting the person that you will be shadowing, compile a few questions to ask them as this will make your meeting far more constructive. The questions could include the following.

- Why did you decide to become a nurse or midwife?

- What nursing/midwifery jobs have you had so far and what did you learn from each?

- What are the benefits and challenges of your current job?

- What are the qualities that you need to be an effective nurse/ midwife?

Experience can help your university application

Most universities recruiting to nursing and midwifery programmes don't insist on prior experience or shadowing but do advise that it helps. In reality, as entry to courses is competitive, such experience often helps a lot, not least because it helps you get a realistic view of the professional field you are applying to. As 50% of the training programme is clinical placement, your university will want to be confident that you have a realistic awareness of the nature of care you will be involved in – you won't learn reality from television hospital drama!

Midwifery

Practising midwives are sometimes inundated with requests for shadowing or experience from aspiring midwifery students; they will not be able to help most enquirers. However, you will probably find that you, family members or friends already know a midwife – this is a relationship to cultivate so that you can ask questions and gain information. You might also offer to support (for free) your local midwifery services, for example by making the refreshments or preparing/clearing rooms used for antenatal classes and then observing the group for their series of meetings.

Children's nursing

Many applicants for children's nursing have some experience of working with healthy children, for example baby sitting or work experience in a nursery. This is certainly helpful, but children's nurses are involved in caring for unwell children and their anxious families. Where possible, it is useful to gain experience with children who do not enjoy normal health. Shadowing in hospital wards for children is occasionally possible, but volunteering for local groups supporting children with additional needs or disability is more widely available: examples include 'opportunity groups', holiday play schemes and riding/activity schemes for disabled children. Children involved in such groups often have more than one health constraint. Volunteering gives you the opportunity to observe needs and to practise core but often particularly complex skills such as communication.

Adult nursing

There are numerous opportunities for gaining experience working with adults who have additional needs – physical, social or emotional. In addition to formal work experience in hospitals or care institutions, considerable insight into the needs of frail or unwell adults can be gained from voluntary work. It is well worth approaching local nursing or residential homes, day centres and support groups (for example for people who have had a stroke). If time allows, a very effective approach is to offer to volunteer for, say, two hours each week, continuing this over a period of time, perhaps for six months or more.

Mental health nursing and learning disability nursing

Formal work experience in hospitals or care institutions is not always straightforward, not least for reasons of confidentiality. However, insight into the needs of people with mental health needs or disabled learning can be gained from voluntary work. Many, perhaps most, nursing homes offer professional nursing care for people with dementia and a wide range of other mental health needs. Similarly, residential settings, sometimes managed by charities or local authorities, offer extended care and home life for local people with learning disabilities. Many such nursing and residential settings greatly appreciate volunteers, who in turn gain insight into the reality of client care. Time permitting, a regular, weekly commitment for six months or more gives volunteers the potential to build an understanding of the duties and roles undertaken in these branches of nursing.

APPLYING TO STUDY NURSING AND MIDWIFERY

Educational qualifications

There are a variety of entry routes into nursing and midwifery for both school/college leavers and mature students. Currently nurses can train on a diploma or degree course in nursing. From 2013 entry to nursing will be by the degree route only and some universities may be offering only this route from September 2011, so you need to check before applying. Entry to midwifery is only through the degree route and application is very competitive.

Anyone wishing to train as a nurse or a midwife needs to have one of the following entry requirements, stipulated by the NMC:

■ five GCSEs at grade C or above or SCEs in English and one science, for entry to the diploma in nursing

■ five GCSEs at grade C or above or SCEs in English, science and maths, for entry to the degree in midwifery

■ universities will expect applicants to have A levels or Scottish Highers for entry to degrees and advanced diplomas in nursing or midwifery. For midwifery, you should have good A level grades in a minimum of two or three subjects including a science such as biology. Many universities will ask for As and Bs. Check the A level or Scottish Higher grades required by each university that you are interested in, using UCAS, as these will vary.

Equivalent qualifications are also accepted:

■ GNVQ intermediate level plus one GCSE, grade A or above, **or** SVQ Level 2

■ GNVQ Advanced level or NVQ Level 3 or SVQ Level 3, GSVQ Level 3

■ Access to Higher Education

■ BTEC National or Higher National Diploma in a care-related discipline

■ passes in Northern Ireland Grammar School Senior Certificate of Education

■ NNEB-awarded qualification from 1985 onwards

■ International Baccalaureate.

The NMC entry requirements offer a wide range of initial routes into nursing and midwifery. As such a wide range of A levels and equivalent qualifications are available to students, it is important to check that your

The School of Nursing and Midwifery at the University of East Anglia

Our School of Nursing and Midwifery is a fantastic place to start your career in nursing. We're passionate about our work and we have an outstanding teaching record – our nursing courses are ranked second in the *Guardian University Guide 2011*. We will encourage and develop your passion and capability in nursing. Our 'research active' culture will nurture your commitment to life-long learning and professional development. You will work in first-class teaching and clinical facilities.

We offer courses in Adult Nursing, Mental Health Nursing, Children's Nursing and Learning Disabilities Nursing, Midwifery and Operating Department Practice. All course fees are paid for by the regional Health Authority and an additional NHS student bursary is also available for other expenses.

Our approach is through 'Evidence Based Learning' – which means it's focused on patient needs and problem solving. Our students think that this, along with the opportunities we arrange for you to get front-line experience from the very early stages of the course, make our courses dynamic and rewarding.

The UEA is a great place at which to 'live and learn', with a unique atmosphere and fantastic opportunities in and beyond your studies; a place where you'll make life-long friendships and develop as a person, fit and capable for your nursing vocation.

Nursing at the University of East Anglia – a student view

Elizabeth Walton is a first year student on a three-year course in Adult Health Nursing at the University of East Anglia. Before choosing the UEA, she took a good look at other nursing schools.

'I researched other courses around the country, but the UEA has such an excellent reputation and it's now number two in the *Guardian* league tables. So it was the obvious choice for me,' she says.

Early patient contact is a key part of the course. 'I was placed on a surgical ward at The Queen Elizabeth Hospital in King's Lynn after two months. It was a fantastic experience and the support and encouragement I received were excellent.'

The focus of the UEA course is Evidence Based Learning, where students work in groups to find solutions to real patient problems. 'It's a great way to learn because we have guidance from expert teachers and we're encouraged to think practically for ourselves' says Elizabeth.

So what does the future hold for Elizabeth? 'There is still so much to learn, but I'm very interested in palliative, end of life care. For the time-being my focus is here – the UEA is a wonderful place to learn and I would recommend it to anyone who wants a career in nursing.'

programme of study is acceptable for entry to undergraduate courses. Candidates studying sciences at A level need to make sure that they are studying biology to the right level, especially for entry to nursing courses at Russell Group universities and all midwifery degree courses. Alternative qualifications, such as the 14–19 Diploma in Sciences, also need to be scrutinised to ensure that they include enough biology and chemistry to be accepted for entry to a higher education nursing or midwifery course. If you are unsure, check with the appropriate university admissions departments to make sure that your A level choices or equivalents meet their entry requirements.

Training routes

For nursing, a student has the option to choose between four specialist branches:

1   adult nursing

2   children's nursing

3   learning disabilities nursing

4   mental health nursing.

Nurses make up the largest group of professionals in the NHS with 400,000 working for the organisation.

(NHS Careers)

There are many differences between these branches, so you need to be sure that you have acquired appropriate knowledge and work experience to prove that you are suitable for a place in your preferred branch.

Nursing diploma and degree courses consist of around 50% theory and 50% practical placements over a three-year full-time course. Placements are an important part of a nurse's training as they underpin and expand on what has been taught in the lecture theatre. They will include placements in a variety of hospital wards, in community health and other health care settings. At some universities students may also get the opportunity to carry out an elective placement.

Postgraduate courses lasting two years are also available for anyone wishing to train as a nurse after completing a first degree, and applications are through UCAS.

Midwifery degrees, like nursing degrees, comprise roughly 50% theoretical training and 50% practical placements. The practical placements underpin and elaborate on what has been taught at university and are essential to the training of a midwife. As with nursing, placements take place in a variety of settings, in hospital and the community.

THE APPLICATION PROCESS

Diploma and degree courses in nursing and midwifery are offered at around 60 universities throughout the UK and 11 institutions in Ireland. Applications to all UK higher level courses are made through the Universities and Colleges Admissions Service (UCAS). Visit www.ucas. com at least a year before applying and start to become familiar with the application process and deadlines. Applicants are allowed to apply

Tips for a successful university application

Universities need to be confident that students who start a course will be able to pass the academic requirements of the programme. In addition to the studying, at degree level or equivalent, you will have assessments, examinations and assignments to complete, all of which must be passed. In setting their entry requirements for each course, universities often publish their minimum grade and subject requirements at least a year ahead of the course starting – and these can change. You should check specific requirements with your preferred universities before you apply; attending an open day is always useful. Although minimum grades are just that – a minimum – it is always worth checking out any specific queries with your universities – for example, if you missed your GCSE English examination through illness but are taking A level humanities subjects, can you still apply?

When choosing universities to apply for there are numerous factors to consider: the quality of the course; distance from home; cost of living; university life; nature of clinical experiences – not forgetting entry requirements. You might want to consider applying for one or two universities with higher entry requirements and one or two that ask for slightly lower grades – this increases your chances of getting an offer that matches your likely examination results.

to a maximum of five institutions, so make sure that you research the institutions that offer nursing or midwifery carefully before completing the online application form. Visit any universities you are considering applying to and use this opportunity to ask questions of staff and students. Don't just find out about the courses: also ask about the clinical placements, the accommodation and the social life. You will be spending three years on your higher education course, so make sure that it suits you. In Ireland applications to universities are made through the Central Applications Office.

Schools and colleges usually have a well-organised UCAS application procedure headed by a member of staff who provides support to applicants throughout the whole process. If you are still in full- or part-time education, make sure that you are aware of the process run by your institution so that you do not miss any relevant sessions.

Applications are made through the UCAS Apply system, the online application process. The first half of the application form requires biographical information and details of your qualifications. Familiarise yourself with the form **before** you fill it in. (See *How to Complete Your UCAS Application 2011 Entry* (Trotman) for detailed information.)

Personal statement

The personal statement is one of the most important sections of the application form. This is where you have to give reasons for applying to your chosen programmes of study. As with any higher education course, applicants to nursing and midwifery have to show their interest and motivation in the personal statement. Your personal statement is where you prove that you deserve a place on your chosen course of study, so make sure that you provide a well-documented and positive picture of your motivations, experiences and capabilities.

When completing your personal statement, make sure that you thoroughly think about what you want to say. Map out your ideas and be prepared to write several drafts before it is complete. Be positive throughout and give reasons why you want to train as a nurse or midwife: what inspired you; how do your A levels or equivalent qualifications link with and support your career ambitions? Remember to mention your achievements, both those linked to your studies and those gained in leisure or voluntary activities. This is also where to highlight relevant work experience and the skills and experiences you have developed.

Once the personal statement is complete, ensure that it is checked for any spelling and grammatical errors. Does the personal statement really reflect who you are? Will the university admissions staff who read it feel the passion and interest that you have for your chosen profession? Ask someone whose opinion you trust to review what you have written so that any glitches can be removed.

As explored in this book, the various areas of nursing and midwifery practice are very different. The admissions team reviewing your application will normally expect to see your whole application directed towards a specific course, e.g. midwifery or adult nursing. If you are unsure of the area of practice to apply for, try to gain some experience to help confirm your choice of course before you apply. It is quite possible that if you prepare a personal statement directed at two courses you will not convince either admissions team of your suitability.

University interviews

Most nursing and midwifery higher education courses conduct face-to-face interviews as part of their assessment process. You do need to prepare in order to achieve a successful outcome.

Once you receive an invitation to attend for further assessment or interview you will find that it will probably be called a selection day and that you will be required to participate in a number of tasks throughout the day. These could include:

- short English and mathematics tests

- group discussion

- group presentation

- informal meeting with current nursing/midwifery students

- interview, generally by two nurses/midwives or lecturers.

The format of selection days is continuously changing. It could in the future include further tasks such as a questionnaire, in which you have to prove your suitability for your chosen course of study by answering questions indicating your interest and others demonstrating your knowledge of nursing or midwifery.

Preparation counts!

Confidence at interview comes from having prepared well. Start by keeping a folder with a copy of your UCAS form and personal statement. Add any health-related articles or articles about current issues in nursing or midwifery in national newspapers that you have read. Keep information about the course and add any questions you would like to ask at interview. Study your folder before the day and be ready to answer questions in the interview.

Consider questions that you might be asked.

- What attracted you to nursing or midwifery?

- What is the role of a nurse/midwife?

- Why are you interested in the course that you have applied to?

- Tell us about a health-related article you have read recently.

- What relevant work experience do you have?

- How will you cope with the academic and clinical demands of this course?

Check all the information you have received from the university so that you know exactly when and where you will need to be on the day. Make sure that you are well organised, set aside any documents that you have been asked to bring and ensure that you sort out your travel arrangements so that you arrive

> Over 150 nursing diploma and degree courses and 44 midwifery degree courses are currently available in the UK.
>
> (UCAS)

on time, and dress smartly. Throughout the day, be polite, attentive and positive. The interview will probably be carried out by a panel of university staff and they will want to see who you really are and what you will bring to your chosen profession, so this is your opportunity to show them. Enjoy the day and try not to worry about nerves – they know that candidates will be nervous and will bear this in mind when making their decisions.

Mature entry to university courses

Nursing and midwifery attract applicants who have already had careers and families. Some applicants have had a positive experience of care that they received or witnessed, and this inspires them to train at a later stage in their lives. It can at times seem a big step to return to studying but the flexible entry routes provide applicants with a variety of initial options for progression on to courses. While it can be a challenging step, students with further life and work experience are welcomed because they bring an added, positive dimension to college and university courses. The NMC specifies a wide range of entry requirements, including Access courses, which have traditionally been favoured by mature students. Access courses are offered by many sixth-form and further education colleges and can be studied on a more flexible basis than full-time courses. In most instances universities are looking for mature applicants to provide evidence of recent academic study – they want to be sure that you will succeed on a degree course. There is no upper age limit in the UK for entry to nursing or midwifery training.

Mature students apply through UCAS in the normal way and can find themselves feeling awkward that their application is 'different' from that of a 17 or 18 year old. Indeed, while most UK students list GCSEs in their application, some applicants may have GCE O levels or CSEs; mature students also often present a diverse range of qualifications from other employment roles, for example accountancy, banking or caring awards. These older or more diverse awards are often accepted by universities, but it is well worth checking with the admissions office or admissions tutor first, perhaps at an open day.

As the university concerned will want to be confident that you can successfully complete the academic components of the course they will often require evidence of recent (within the last five years) study to Level 3 (GCE A level) standard. For mature students, undertaking an A level is time consuming – generally two years. However, many further education colleges offer Access to Higher Education courses, which are specifically designed for mature students whose academic skills need updating before they go to university. These courses are widely accepted by universities (but check carefully with your preferred institutions). You should aim for an Access course intended for those wanting to progress to health professional courses – typical subjects include human biology or biology, psychology or sociology and health studies, and may include other options such as English language. You will also need evidence of examined competence in mathematics – normally GCSE or O level Mathematics with at least grade C or CSE grade 1. Other qualifications may be considered, including Level 2 or 3 Numeracy – there are many other equivalents, so you are strongly advised to check with your preferred universities well before you apply. It is worth noting that there can be considerable variation in entry requirements between universities, and these may be modified further for mature applicants on the basis of other demonstrable skills.

Learn with the best: Providing the nurses and midwives of the future

The University of Southampton, Faculty of Health Sciences is leading the way in nursing and midwifery, offering:

- cutting edge, research led teaching
- exciting and varied practise experiences
- virtual interactive practice suites for a realistic learning experience
- excellent staff student ratios
- supportive and friendly environment

The Faculty of Health Sciences is proud to be forward thinking and innovative in delivering high quality teaching. It is currently ranked top in England and third in the UK according to *The Times Good University Guide 2010*, which uses many factors including research funding and student surveys to create the list.

Student story

I never believed that University was something I could ever contemplate undertaking.

I had heard of the amazing opportunities the University of Southampton offered and knew they were **renowned for their courses in Nursing and Midwifery**, (amongst many others) as well as their exceptional facilities, social prospects and excellent teaching.

After further research into the course and the University itself, I discovered the **amazing support and services** Southampton offered. With a vast range of financial guidance provided by Student Services, they not only offer a number of options to help students finance their courses, they provide advice in managing money and answer any concerns you may have. This combined with the **outstanding academic support** from an immeasurable number of sources and the fantastic opportunities presented from a **thriving social life** have led to an incredible University experience.

I have studied hard, managed financially and made friends for life. I am now, amongst other things, student representative and student buddy to first years and aim to offer them the same brilliant experience that I was given.

After three unforgettable years of studying, I am currently preparing to qualify as a Registered Nurse in Adult Nursing with clear goals, objectives and a wealth of career prospects.

Contact details

Faculty of Health Sciences
Nightingale Building (Building 67)
University of Southampton
Highfield
Southampton
Hampshire
United Kingdom
SO17 1BJ

Website: www.southampton.ac.uk/healthsciences/
Email: HealthSciences@soton.ac.uk
Phone: 023 8059 5500
Fax: 023 8059 7900
Join us on Facebook at www.facebook.com/SouthamptonUni. HealthSciences

As a mature applicant it is well worth doing an analysis of the skills, talents, experience and qualifications you can offer – from all sources since adolescence. This can substantially help your thinking as you prepare an application.

It is also worth seeking support for writing your personal statement for UCAS – either from a college tutor or perhaps a health professional you work with.

Applying as a mature student: your questions answered

Am I too old to start nurse training?

There is no upper age limit in the UK for entry to nursing or midwifery training.

Will I have to work any night shifts?

Students normally work many of their practice hours on the same shift as their supporting mentor. There is also a requirement to experience the full 24-hour pattern of care. All students will work some early starts, late finishes, nights and weekends. However, it is frequently possible to plan shifts well in advance, for example to accommodate occasional family events or a partner's employment pattern. It is not possible to arrange shifts around school times.

Will childcare facilities be available?

Probably, but it may be awkward as you will spend 20–24 weeks a year at university and 20–24 weeks a year in practice. Either of these settings may well offer childcare facilities but they may not necessarily open for early starts or late finishes. Most parents find independent arrangements are best; most areas have childminders available for the unusual hours of placement; Sure Start advisers should be able to help.

Will childcare be free?

No. You will need to pay the going rates. However, if you are entitled to an NHS bursary payment you may be able to reclaim part or all of these costs.

Is anything free?

All full-time students (and this is particularly relevant to mature students) are entitled to a discount on their local authority council tax. Many councils give 100% exemption; if another adult lives in the same house your share will be discounted. Additionally, at the time of writing, all UK, EU and EEA residents have their tuition fees paid for studying nursing or midwifery at UK universities.

What if my children are unwell? Can I take time off?

There are fixed requirements for nursing and midwifery courses; any time missed will need to be 'made up'. However, universities will be sympathetic to your circumstances; it is essential to contact your tutors as soon as the problem arises.

Will I have to travel far from home?

This will vary according to the university, but for most people there will be an element of travel to placements. These can be some distance away – up to 30 or 40 miles at some institutions – so check with your preferred universities. Your university may take account of your circumstances, access to transport, etc. – again, check carefully before you apply. If you are entitled to an NHS bursary excess travel costs to placement may be reclaimable.

Will I be too old to get a job afterwards?

A straightforward answer – no!

Will my experience as a care worker be helpful?

Definitely yes – you will have a realistic insight into the roles and demands of health care. But you will still need to meet the academic entry criteria of the university.

FEES AND FUNDING

Residents of the UK, EU and EEA are exempt from the tuition fee charges made by universities. In addition, UK residents studying nursing or midwifery at UK universities may receive a bursary to support them while they are at university; for some courses, including all degree programmes, the bursary is means tested. Further information on the exact amount can be obtained from individual universities or the NHS Student Grants Unit. The NHS can sometimes offer secondments to staff who have been in post for over 12 months and this is worth investigating further if you are already working for the NHS in a Level 1 to 4 occupation. A seconded student will normally receive basic pay from the NHS but not a bursary, and may be expected to go back to work for the NHS trust that has seconded them.

ARMED FORCES NURSES

The British Army, Royal Air Force and Royal Navy all recruit student nurses, sponsor them while they undertake their university degree course and subsequently employ them on completion of their studies. Entry into these positions is competitive, as many people are keen to take on the forces lifestyle with the accompanying benefits and challenges. Applicants currently need to have a minimum of 240 UCAS points at AS/A level, Scottish Higher or equivalents, and GCSEs or equivalents including English language, maths and a science at grade C or above. Applicants also have to be committed and enthusiastic team players who can remain calm but react quickly in emergencies. All three forces presently train student nurses at one university, and initial applications can be made by visiting your local Armed Forces Careers Information Office.

As a forces student nurse, before commencing your studies you will have to complete a period of basic military training, which introduces you to leadership and military skills. Once qualified you will be assigned a rotational nursing post for your first year, providing you with a variety of health care environments to work in, including medical, surgical and acute settings.

As a forces registered nurse you will be providing support to both military staff and civilians and will be working both in the UK and overseas. The work will be rewarding and challenging, due to the responsibilities that you will be required to take on and the countries that you will work in around the world.

SUMMARY

Applications to nursing or midwifery courses are not straightforward. This chapter has attempted to show how you can make yourself a worthy candidate by getting the right type of work experience and attaining the general skills and academic qualifications required by universities. The intricacies of the application process and possible sources of funding have also been highlighted, along with what could happen in the university interview. Success in all these areas should translate into a number of offers on nursing or midwifery courses, followed by a fascinating three years in higher education on your preferred course of study. The time will no doubt fly by and before you know it you will be turning your attention to applying for your first job as a professional nurse or midwife.

Chapter Ten

HOW TO FIND YOUR FIRST ROLE

Although student nurses and midwives have already decided on the professions that they wish to enter after graduation, they still need to apply for employment. Clinical placements give first-hand experience of the type of employment that most students will be entering, but there are a number of further steps that have to be taken to make the transition from education to employment.

THE APPLICATION PROCESS

When you apply for employment you will be working through a process consisting of a number of stages. The first stage is centred on you – even before you start to complete an application form you will need to think about who you are and assess your skills. Everyone is unique so it is important that you pick out your strengths and interests in order to match yourself to the right vacancies. This will also help you to consider the areas of nursing or midwifery that you are most interested in.

Skills and experiences

Your formal nursing or midwifery training will have provided you with many skills and experiences that you can use to prove that you are capable of succeeding in your chosen career. This is not, however, the only area of your life in which you have developed skills and been successful. Before beginning the application process it is useful to step back, assess your skills and find evidence of where and how you have used them. Your skills can come from several areas of your life, for example:

■ your degree or diploma course – both your academic study and your clinical placements

■ current and past employment

■ volunteering

■ clubs and societies – both at university and at home

■ travel – especially any trips that you have organised independently

■ achievements such as Duke of Edinburgh's Award scheme or Young Enterprise.

Skills audit

A skills audit is a tool that can be used to pull together your skills and experiences in order to collect suitable evidence that can be used to inform employers that you are a suitable candidate.

When considering your skills, really think about what you can do. Ask yourself three questions.

1 What am I good at and why?

2 What do I enjoy doing?

3 Where have I recently succeeded and why?

The information you use in your skills audit needs to be robust – it can be used throughout the application process. It is a way of establishing your strengths and experiences, which can be transferred into a CV or application form.

When you are invited to interview you can return to the skills audit to remind yourself of your skills; what they are and where and how you used each one. It can also be revised and used when answering interview questions.

A typical skills audit

Experience	Skill	Evidence
Degree in nursing	Good time manager	I keep a diary to ensure that assignments are completed on time. When on placement I keep a daily 'to do' list to help me carry out my duties.
	Effective team member	I enjoy being part of a multidisciplinary team. In a surgical ward I was able to suggest a way to support a nervous patient who was anxious about their operation. My ideas were listened to and used to support the patient.
Care worker – The Beeches Care Home	Flexible worker	One evening I was helping a resident with her meal when another resident collapsed. I stopped what I was doing and explained to the lady I was helping why I had to leave her temporarily. I went to the other resident's aid, called for assistance and supported my senior colleague until further help arrived and I then went back to my initial task.
University hockey club	Resilience	I regularly play in the ladies' first team and this means attending training sessions on a weekly basis, regardless of the weather.
Independent travel to Europe	Using initiative	On one occasion I had to rebook my accommodation in Italy as the hostel that I was due to stay in was over-booked. I had to identify other hostels, contact the ones that were suitable and book a room for that evening.

FINDING VACANCIES

There are many websites and magazines that you can use when seeking your first professional post.

NHS: www.jobs.nhs.uk

Although the NHS's website advertises the majority of vacancies held in the organisation, there are also other places to look. When you are on placement it is worth looking at noticeboards where you are based in case any vacancies are advertised there.

Professional organisations

The Royal College of Nursing and the Royal College of Midwives advertise vacancies both on their websites and in the professional magazines that go out to members. Their websites are:

■ www.rcnbulletinjobs.co.uk

■ http://jobs.midwives.co.uk.

The nursing and midwifery press

If you are seeking employment in or outside the NHS, either in the UK or overseas, it is useful to look in the many specialist magazines aimed at health care professionals:

■ *Nursing Times* (www.nursingtimes.net)

■ *Nursing Standard* (http://nursingstandard.rcnpublishing.co.uk)

■ *British Journal of Midwifery* (www.britishjournalofmidwifery.com).

Employment agencies

There are many employment agencies advertising part-time and full-time vacancies. If you are seeking employment in the NHS it is worthwhile visiting NHS Professionals, the NHS's recruitment site for flexible workers: www.nhsprofessionals.nhs.uk.

Outside the NHS, towns and cities across the UK have agencies that recruit health care professionals. Details of these companies can be found in local newspapers and in directories such as the *Yellow Pages*.

National and local newspapers

The press still remains a source of vacancy information. If you are looking for a job that is a little more unusual, look in newspapers for ideas. National newspapers advertise jobs: the *Guardian* advertises health vacancies on Wednesdays and they can also be found at www. guardianjobs.co.uk.

Local newspapers may advertise vacancies in care homes or GPs' surgeries. If you are committed to staying locally start reviewing the jobs pages of your neighbourhood paper on a weekly basis. You will also be able to look at these vacancies by going to the paper's website.

Local authorities

Local authorities also advertise nursing vacancies online. Look at your local council's website: you should be able to search their vacancies pages.

Networks and contacts

Having undertaken a vocational course you will have met nursing and midwifery staff who will be able to inform you of suitable vacancies. If you have enjoyed working in a certain department it is worth asking the ward or section manager if there might be suitable vacancies in the near future. You can leave a current CV and/or contact details so that you can be informed of any positions that arise.

COMPETITIVE JOBS

Many student nurses and midwives have one or two clinical departments that they wish to work in when they have qualified. If you are interested in working in a department which is competitive to enter, it can be useful to build up your experience by working in that environment as a health care assistant while you are still a student. Some students also organise a further placement in the area that they wish to eventually work in, to give them an edge when applying for vacancies.

Nurses and midwives who want to work overseas once they have qualified are usually expected to have at least one year's post-qualification employment experience.

FIRST PROFESSIONAL JOB

Most newly qualified nurses and midwives start their professional careers in the NHS at Level 5. These posts can sometimes be rotational, giving you the opportunity to work in a variety of specialisms over a set number of months. The benefit of this is that you will gain an insight into a variety of clinical areas before you finally opt for a permanent location.

This is not, however, always the case: some newly qualified staff will go straight into departments or wards that were advertised as a Level 5 post.

YOUR CV

A good CV is a valuable way of showing an employer that you have a range of skills and experience that will complement their current workforce. A CV is a marketing tool that can secure you an interview, so it is worth taking time over writing it. Many organisations, including the NHS, expect you to complete an application form when you apply for nursing or midwifery employment, but you should have an up-to-date CV when you are embarking on finding a new job, for several reasons.

- **Speculative applications:** you may know exactly where you wish to work but there is no vacancy there. Send in your CV to inform the ward manager that you are interested in working in that department.

- **Careers fairs:** leave a copy of your CV with employers you talk to at careers fairs. If they are interested in you they may contact you.

- **Niche employment areas:** you may be interested in a specialist field of nursing or midwifery; sending your CV to these departments or organisations is one way of showing your interest.

- **Strengthening your application:** a well-constructed CV can help you to fill in application forms. The CV will provide you with key ideas and evidence that you can expand on in a personal statement and at interview.

- **Maintaining your portfolio:** your CV can go at the front of your portfolio and be taken to interviews so that recruiters can easily see what skills and experience you have.

CVs are written in a variety of formats, from a one-page outline to a two-page skills-based format. As a newly qualified nurse or midwife you need to write a CV that really shows employers what you have experienced over the length of your training. Other areas of your life also need to be incorporated into your CV: this will provide a complete picture of your experience and capabilities. Employers read many CVs, so put your information on two sides of good-quality A4 paper. Provide more information about your most relevant experience and be concise about other areas of your life. If you have had other careers before starting your training you need to give this information succinctly.

Although you will have a prototype CV, every copy that is sent out should be tailored to the needs and requirements of the specific employer. If you are applying for an advertised vacancy, ensure that your CV meets the requirements for the post. These are included in the job description and person specification for each vacancy. Employers will want to see that you have tailored your CV to their vacancy and they will not need to have information that does not match what they are seeking.

Writing a CV

For a nursing or midwifery CV to be truly effective it needs to be balanced in favour of your academic and clinical experience.

The first page of your CV really needs to show your passion and interest in nursing and midwifery through a clear and focused explanation of your academic training and related clinical experience. After providing your personal contact details, you could capture the main messages that you are trying to convey in the CV in a 'personal profile' or 'career objectives' section. Follow this with your professional education and qualifications, with information on your nursing or midwifery degree or diploma, including critical dates – when you qualified and received your PIN. The rest of page one should highlight the various clinical placements that you have had, under the sub-heading 'Professional skills and experience' – this will give the employer a good understanding of what you have done. Include four or more of your placements in this section and try to present a general picture of what you learned in each of these settings – without repeating yourself. When deciding what to include, think of three to five points that illustrate any new procedures that you developed in each setting, plus any new ways of working or successes that you experienced.

Page two of your CV will illustrate the rest of your experience, including your previous general education, work experience, additional skills and interests.

Sample CV

Your name
University or home address
Telephone number(s) (land line and mobile)
Email
Date of birth (optional)

Personal profile

Two to three sentences explaining who you are and where you are studying. Mention a few of your skills. The area of nursing or midwifery that you wish to enter.

Professional education and qualifications

Sept 2007–Sept 2010	Name of university
	Course title
Date of registration	Registered Nurse/Midwife
	PIN – to be advised

Professional skills and experience

June 2009–Sept 2009   Surgical Unit, Any Town Hospital

Three or four bullet points explaining the duties and responsibilities that you had whilst on your placement.

- duty 1   ■ responsibilities 1
- duty 2   ■ responsibilities 2

Oct 2008–Nov 2008   Community Care Unit, Any Town PCT

- Follow the same pattern as above. Remember to highlight any points that were particularly important about each individual placement.
- Use this format to explain the majority of your clinical placements. Less information may be given on the first two placements undertaken.

General education

Sept 2004–June 2006   Eastern College
3 A levels: Biology (B), Psychology (B), English (B)

Sept 1999–June 2004   Western High School
7 GCSEs at A–C, including English, Maths and Double Science.

Work experience

Nov 2006–June 2009   NHS Professionals
Health care assistant

■ Explain duties and the skills acquired in this post.
■ Aim for three to four bullet points.

Sept 2004–May 2006   Sainsbury's
Sales assistant

■ Succinct and informative points explaining duties undertaken and skills acquired.
■ Aim for three to four bullet points.

Additional skills and interests

■ Relevant training courses attended and dates.
■ IT – mention packages that you use.
■ Full, clean driving licence.
■ Student member of the Royal College of Nurses/Midwives.

University netball club   Member of the netball team.
Regularly attend training sessions.

Swimming   Regularly swim for relaxation

References

Dr A. B. Case   Mrs B Harriott
Lecturer   Senior Sister
University of Hightown   Surgical Unit
School of Nursing   Anytown Hospital
and Midwifery   Anytown Road
Northfield   Any Town
Hightown   AO12 8BG
HT3 1HG

Also include telephone number and email if available.

Complete the CV by adding two referees who can give a good account of your capabilities. At the start of your nursing or midwifery career, one referee should be your personal tutor; the second could be someone who has recently supervised you on a clinical placement.

COVERING LETTER

The majority of CVs, especially if they are speculative, should be accompanied by a covering letter. The covering letter is an opportunity to introduce yourself to an employer and to explain why you are writing. It also gives you an opportunity to provide further details about your most relevant skills and experience.

If you are applying by email you should send your covering letter and CV as two attachments. The email will act as a focused introduction.

As with a CV, the covering letter needs to be concise – one page of four to five paragraphs is enough.

When you send a targeted covering letter to a nursing or midwifery employer, you are not only introducing your CV but also highlighting a number of points, such as:

- your interest in and knowledge of their organisation, hospital or ward
- a sample of the range of relevant nursing or midwifery experience and skills that you bring.

Your covering letter should whet the employer's interest and make them want to read your CV and – hopefully – invite you for an interview.

APPLICATION FORMS AND ONLINE APPLICATIONS

Online applications are now the most common way of applying for nursing and midwifery vacancies in the UK. The NHS jobs website includes a standard application form that you set up and can modify every time you apply for a vacancy. Other employers will use similar recruitment systems and only a small number of organisations may ask for a letter of application, CV or a stand-alone application. When completing an online application form it is worthwhile not adding large sections of information straight into the form. Sections such as the personal statement and information about previous jobs can first be written in Word and then pasted into the form.

Application forms follow a similar layout to CVs. The first third asks you for personal biographical details, including your name, address and qualifications. Take care when completing the form – make sure, for example that you give a professional-sounding email address, as this may well be the way in which the employer, especially the NHS, will maintain contact with you. The second section will ask for details about your previous employers, your duties and responsibilities. This section needs to include the key points about each job you have had. While it should be concise, it also needs to include the duties and responsibilities you have had – this provides an insight into your employment history.

Personal statement

Application forms include a section where you are asked to give reasons why you wish to be considered for the post. This section is known as the supporting evidence section or the personal statement.

Employers will match the evidence provided in a personal statement to the person specification that has been compiled for a vacancy. Anyone meeting the essential criteria set out in a person specification should be invited for interview. All applicants will have access to the job description and person specification for a vacancy and the trick is to prove that you have the skills and experience set out in these documents. This is predominantly done by marketing your relevant evidence in your personal statement.

The personal statement is therefore crucial to the success of your application and has to be carefully constructed. Bear the following points in mind.

■ Start with a strong and positive first paragraph. What inspired you to become a nurse or midwife and why are you interested in this vacancy?

- Show your interest in the employer you are applying to. Give one or two points saying why you want to work for them. If you carried out a placement with them, why did you enjoy it and what did you learn about the ward or unit when you were with them?

- Give evidence to prove that you have the skills that they are seeking for in this vacancy. Much of your evidence will come from your clinical placements, but you can use examples from other areas of your life.

- What have you gained from your academic study? How do you keep up to date with new ideas in your profession? How do you wish to further your professional knowledge in the future?

- Are you aware of professional codes of conduct, the importance of clinical governance and evidence-based practice?

- Mention leisure interests, voluntary work and membership of clubs and societies. This shows that you are multi-faceted. It also shows that you have ways of relaxing after a stressful day at work.

Although there is no optimum length, you do need to keep this section focused and factual, so aim to produce a personal statement that is around a page and a half long.

Make sure that you can substantiate everything in the statement – you may be asked to expand on certain points at interview.

Check your spelling and grammar – a badly written personal statement will not be well received. Ask someone else to review what you have written.

Other information

The rest of the application form will require you to give truthful answers about your health and any disabilities. If you do have a disability it is always best to make employers aware of this as they will then be able to provide any necessary support required.

Sections dealing with issues such as criminal convictions must also be answered truthfully and accurately. If you are working for the NHS you will have to undergo a further check by the Criminal Records Bureau, so any points that have not been mentioned will come to light at a later stage.

References

You will need to give two referees who can substantiate what you
have said in your application. One should be your personal tutor at
university and another could be someone from one of your recent clinical
placements, such as a supervisor. Always ask their permission first so
that they know they are likely to receive requests for references.

Finally ...

Make sure that all sections have been accurately completed before you
send off your application form.

INTERVIEWS AND ASSESSMENT CENTRES

Invitations to attend a job interview are usually sent out two or three
weeks after the closing date has passed. Many organisations now use
email to invite candidates to interview, so keep an eye on your in-box to
make sure that you do not miss any correspondence. The information
you receive will explain what will happen during the interview and whether
you will be expected to participate in any other tasks, such as a group
discussion. Further recruitment tasks are now being used by hospitals,
including several in London and other cities in the UK – you could, for
example, be required to take a drugs calculation test. Be prepared.

When you receive the invitation to an interview, start by congratulating
yourself. Your application will have been measured against the criteria
set out in the person specification and you have met or exceeded what
is required, so this is a successful step forward in the process. You also
need to confirm that you will be attending the interview.

Assessment centres

Hospital trusts, especially in large cities such as London, use assessment
centres as part of their recruitment procedure. If invited to an assessment
centre you will have to undergo a number of short tests and probably
also be interviewed on the day or soon after.

Selecting candidates through the use of assessment centres is seen
by many employers as a fair and objective way of recruiting staff. This
is because objective measures of an individual's performance are being

observed and assessed, and this gives the employer more than the interview as a recruitment tool.

Assessment centres are used to assess your suitability for a post using a number of techniques such as:

■ group discussion

■ objective structured clinical examination test

■ written paper

■ drugs calculation test.

When you are invited to attend an assessment centre you will be informed about the activities that you will be participating in. As in the rest of the application process, throughout your time at an assessment centre you will be measured against the competencies for the post that you have applied to.

How to prepare

Go back to the job description and person specification for the post and ensure that you know what type of person the employer is intending to recruit. Make sure that you know what competencies are being sought (check the person specification): these are the ones that candidates will be assessed against at the assessment centre. Ensure that you are aware of current issues associated with the vacancy or the trust.

A few tips for the day of the assessment/interview:

■ get plenty of rest the night before

■ arrive on time

■ be yourself

■ try to stay calm

■ follow instructions and ask for clarification if they are not clear

■ be aware of any time constraints and keep to them

■ make sure that you take part in any discussions, but don't dominate them

■ be positive and enthusiastic

■ remember that you are being assessed at all times, so make sure that you are behaving appropriately.

Interview preparation

Success at interview is usually down to good preparation. When you write an assignment or sit an exam, you prepare and research beforehand. An interview needs the same amount of preparation – this will instil confidence in you and will give you a greater chance of success.

Before the day, go back to your application and read what you wrote. Read information about the hospital or organisation that you have applied to – what do you know about them and are there any initiatives or successes that they are involved in? Be aware of any relevant national health care documents that are of importance to the role you have applied for. Have an understanding of current health care issues that are being discussed in the media. If you read a quality newspaper three or four times a week you should maintain an insight into the major health care issues of the day.

Although many workplaces are very busy it is useful to visit the ward or unit that you have applied to work in. Contact the relevant person to see if this can be organised and use the opportunity to ask questions and see what the working environment is like.

Before the day, plan your journey and make sure that you know where the interview will be held. Even if you have had one of your clinical placements in the hospital where you have been invited to interview, you may not know the specific part of the building where you will be seen, so ensure that you know where you are going. Public places like hospitals are very busy during the day, so leave yourself plenty of time to park if you will be arriving by car.

Make sure that you know what will be required of you on the interview day. Will you only be attending for the interview or will there be other activities that you will also be expected to do? Have you been asked to bring along any further information such as your portfolio? (If you have, the panel will ask to see it, usually at the end of the interview.)

Portfolios are usually A4 document folders that hold 12–15 pieces of critical evidence that back up what you have included in your application form and CV. If you are compiling a portfolio, start by including a contents page and follow this with your current CV, copies of placement reports, educational certificates and any other documents that you wish to highlight, including letters or commendations from clinical and academic staff or patients.

Practise answering interview questions. This can be done with friends from your course; or you might be able to arrange a mock interview with a member of your university's academic staff. Ask your tutors or careers service for sample questions and go online – many are now posted on the web. Mock interviews are also offered by many university careers services, so find out if they are available and book one to help you prepare for your interview. As you and your fellow students start going to interviews, try to remember the questions that you have been asked and share them so that you can become more proficient with your answers.

Prepare three or four questions to ask at the end of your interview. It is useful to have these prepared in advance as you may not be able to think of any suitable questions on the actual day. Areas that you might wish to find out more about could include what your first month in the job would consist of and the training that you will receive in your first year.

The interview

Attending an interview can feel challenging, but remember, it is your skills and experience as a nurse or midwife that are being assessed, not you as an individual. The interview is also a chance for you to decide if you like the hospital or trust and the vacancy that you have applied for.

How you behave at interview plays an important part in your overall success on the day, so bear the following points in mind.

Dress smartly

Once you secure your first nursing or midwifery job you will probably be wearing a uniform, but at interview you will be expected to be smartly dressed.

Be composed

Be positive and professional throughout the interview – everything you say and do will be observed by others. Shake hands if this is offered and take your seat once it is indicated.

Speech and eye contact

Smile and maintain good eye contact when you are in the interview. Try not to worry about nerves and do not let them overpower you. The interviewers know that candidates may be a little nervous. Remember, they are comparing you to the person specification and they really want to find out more about what you can do.

Getting stuck

If you do not fully hear a question, ask for it to be repeated. Take a deep breath before answering questions, especially if they are tricky ones.

Any further questions?

You will have an opportunity near the end of the interview to ask your prepared questions.

After the interview

After your interview, you should be told when you will hear if you have been successful. If this does not happen, make sure to ask when you are invited to ask further questions.

For more advice on interview techniques see *You're Hired! Interview: Tips & Techniques for a Brilliant Interview*, published by Trotman.

The application process is complicated and this chapter has outlined the various stages that you will work through when applying for your first nursing or midwifery post. The importance of identifying your relevant skills and experiences was outlined, as well as how these can be used when writing your CV, covering letters and applications. To maximise your chances of success at interview you have to be well prepared and this too has been highlighted, along with how to tackle assessment centres, which are now being used by a number of health care employers. Once you get your first professional job you will be starting a chapter in your employment history and in two or three years you may start to think about how you move on beyond your Level 5 or 6 post into a more senior nursing or midwifery post.

Helen Pearson, BN(Hons) Paediatric Nursing, RSCN

I qualified in 2006 with an Advanced Diploma in Paediatric Nursing and initially I undertook a sabbatical year working at Southampton University before applying for nursing posts. I started to look for nursing jobs to commence in the autumn of 2007 and after the applications I initially submitted I was unsuccessful in getting to interview.

Nursing is a competitive world and I knew employers would be looking through many applications and therefore I needed mine to stand out from the crowd. With the help of the careers service I was able to write my supporting information statement that highlighted my strengths, supported with examples from both my student nurse experience and extra-curricular activities. I was extremely involved with university life, from being societies officer of the students' union to president of the Nursing and Midwifery Society. I learnt valuable life skills from my extra-curricular activities and believed it showed potential employers that I created opportunities for myself and was a team player. Life is about having a good work–life balance; nursing can be stressful and employers are keen to see what employees participate in outside their working life.

Applying for my first job was an exciting time with mixed emotions but I believe the key to being successful lies in the supporting information statement. Highlight your strengths, be factual and, most important, add a sentence as to why you want to work for that particular hospital: this shows you have done your research into the area you're applying to.

Chapter Eleven
CAREER PROGRESSION AND FUTURE PROSPECTS

The health care professions are constantly developing and changing and anyone working in nursing or midwifery will soon see that there are many opportunities available to them once they have worked for (usually) two years after qualification.

The exciting thing is that the way your career develops is down to the choices that you make. You may wish to consolidate your training and further develop certain skills in specific clinical settings. Alternatively, you may wish to progress into senior managerial posts or gain further academic qualifications. The choice is yours and it has to be factored into the lifestyle you wish to maintain and the responsibilities you already have.

Your first year in employment, after gaining registration, will be a busy and rewarding time. Make time to keep a reflective log or diary capturing what you have learned and what skills and experience you wish to develop. Use the following headings to guide and collect your thoughts.

- What skills have I learned?

- What experience do I wish to capture?

- What skills and experience do I wish to develop?

- How can they be developed?

Use this information when discussing your future training needs and career plans when you meet with your line manager as the year progresses.

Formal education does not stop once you have completed your first degree or diploma in either profession. The NMC stipulates that in order to remain on their register, all nurses and midwives have to meet the council's post-registration and practice standards (PREP). The standards are there to 'safeguard the health and wellbeing of the public by ensuring that anyone renewing their registration has undertaken a minimum amount of practice' (NMC, *The PREP Handbook*, 2005). In order to maintain their NMC registration, nurses and midwives are expected to have practised for a minimum of 450 hours during the three years prior to the renewal of their registration. The PREP standard also stipulates that 35 hours' (or the equivalent of five days') continuing professional development is undertaken during the three years prior to renewal of registration. You must also keep a personal professional profile or portfolio of the learning activities you have been involved in.

Nurses and midwives begin their first post with a period of preceptorship, similar to a probationary period, which lasts for the first few months of employment. During this time new staff receive supervision and support to ease them into their new roles. During the preceptorship period, for example, nurses are required to develop a number of clinical competencies including handling blood products and cannulation. General competencies are also developed in areas such as leadership, communication and conflict resolution techniques. Once the preceptorship has been completed, you will be very much part of the workforce on your ward or department, as you will have shown that you are a competent practitioner.

SALARIES

The majority of new nurses and midwives begin their career by working in the NHS. As one of the largest employers in the UK, the NHS has clearly defined pay bands for all its directly employed staff, with the exception of doctors, dentists and some very senior managers. The Agenda for Change pay system sets out the salary grades for posts and these are matched to the abilities and responsibilities that a nurse or midwife has developed in their work role. New nurses and midwives enter their professions at Level 5 in the NHS and may progress beyond the starting point of this entry band once they have had their first appraisal, part way through their first year. The NHS has a clearly defined set of key skills that are part of the Knowledge and Skills Framework, for each of its work roles, and staff receive a personal development review annually with their line manager where they are required to give evidence to prove that they are developing and meeting the core and specific dimensions assigned to their post. An annual development plan is also constructed for each member of staff. If satisfactory progress has been made when the plan is reviewed at the end of the year, the individual concerned should receive an incremental rise in their salary. Nurses and midwives entering the profession in 2010 can earn a minimum of £21,176 in the NHS. There are also other benefits, such as a high cost area supplement for those working in inner London – between £4,036 and £6,217. Current NHS pay bands can be viewed at www.nhscareers.nhs.uk/list/payandbenefits.

Nurses and midwives working in the private sector immediately after registration will find that large private health care organisations such as BUPA often match entry-level NHS salaries.

A wide variety of other private sector career opportunities also exist for nurses and midwives and salaries will differ according to the vacancy, so it is important to check the pay and conditions package on offer with every health care vacancy that looks appealing.

CAREER DEVELOPMENT

The 21st century will see many changes and new demands in health care, both in the UK and overseas. In order to meet these changes new career opportunities are developing for nurses and midwives, in both the public and the private sector. Opportunities are available not only in the NHS but also in schools, universities, prisons, the armed forces, care homes, charities, on ocean liners and more.

The NHS offers a wide range of settings that nurses and midwives can work in – hospitals are only one of the options on offer. Factors such as an ageing population and the treatment of long-term conditions such as diabetes in the community mean that the focus is changing to providing nursing care away from hospitals. Nurses and midwives are now taking up more roles in the community in GPs' practices, walk-in centres and schools. District nurses and health visitors are also in demand as hospital stays become shorter and more clinical care is provided in the home. Health promotion has also grown in importance in the UK, with nurses and midwives encouraging healthy lifestyles to help prevent the onset of illnesses.

Beyond Level 5

Eighteen months to two years after registration, many professionals start thinking about career progression. When you reach this point you need to consider where your career interests lie. You need to start deciding, for example, whether you wish to focus more on the clinical side of nursing or midwifery or want to undertake a more managerial post. You may want to get more involved in the education of others or perhaps you like the idea of working in research and helping to develop new treatments and new ways of supporting patients. These functions can be combined within a career, or a greater emphasis can be given to one function, such as management. How you decide to climb the career ladder is a decision that only you can make. You might decide that you will seek promotion every two to three years or that you will continue to develop your clinical and interpersonal skills at a pace dictated by you and your lifestyle.

The NHS Career Framework encourages the individual development and progression of staff. Workforce roles are assigned to the following levels:

- Level 5: Practitioner

- Level 6: Senior practitioner

- Level 7: Advanced practitioner

- Level 8: Consultant practitioner

- Level 9: Senior leader.

Level 6 is usually achieved by nurses and midwives two years after registration. Progression to Level 6 can be achieved through proving competence in a role by meeting the key skills competencies set out in Level 5. Level 6 can also be reached through promotion to the role of senior staff nurse or midwife and thus gaining a number of new responsibilities.

Experienced nursing posts

Level 7, 8 and 9 posts in the NHS include further responsibilities, including managerial, advanced clinical, research or educational responsibilities. Managerial careers include those of the modern matron in a hospital where the post holder has many responsibilities that allow her/him to be highly visible to patients while also being a managerial and clinical professional who is responsible for the management of a group of wards. The role of the modern matron also includes leading and developing the staff team and improving hospital cleanliness through maintaining links with cleaning staff. Other aspects of this post include supporting patients and their families by being highly visible and resolving conflicts. Modern matrons also have the responsibility of empowering nurses by supporting them to improve and develop their nursing practice. There are similar roles in primary care – community matrons and community team leaders.

While this is a many-layered post, it allows anyone with several years' experience and lots of motivation to be involved in a managerial capacity with a variety of health care professionals and others, including nurses, doctors, hospital managers and patients.

Advanced clinical job roles are also available for those interested in specialising in the care of patients with specific illnesses. Nurses undertaking these roles are required to have further specialist knowledge and skills in specific clinical areas. The roles include leading in the treatment of defined patient groups, so empathy, communication and education skills are also important. Job titles in this sector include:

- clinical nurse specialist
- advanced nurse practitioner
- nurse consultant
- health visitor
- community mental health nurse
- consultant health visitor
- school nurse.

Working in medical research

Research is an area of clinical employment that sometimes gets forgotten by nurses and midwives, but they may have enjoyed using research skills at university. There are careers in research in hospitals, universities and with businesses allied to the health service, such as pharmaceutical companies. Research and clinical trials nurses at Levels 7 and 8 investigate clinical areas and help to develop new treatments and protocols. Nurses applying for research posts are expected to have good clinical skills, an enquiring mind and a keenness to discover new protocols and procedures. Anyone who is methodical, well organised and enjoys work that requires you to be precise and attentive to detail should not rule out careers in research.

Working in education

Education plays an important role in the development and upskilling of the existing workforce. It is also crucial to the future growth of the health care sector in the UK. Careers exist for those wishing to train new entrants to either profession in universities and with the NHS. There are lecturer practitioner and lecturer roles at Levels 7 and 8 and university dean and professorial roles at Level 9. Along with clinical skills, jobs in higher education require you to have good interpersonal skills because you will be talking to students individually and also delivering lectures to groups. You will need to be self-motivated, well organised and to enjoy research. You could be expected to write articles and publications, so you will need to enjoy writing and presenting your work to colleagues.

Experienced midwifery posts

Midwives can work in a variety of settings and many remain in hospitals while others move into the community and work in GP practices, charities and children's centres. Many jobs are also integrated, which means that post holders spend time working in the community and in a hospital setting. The first year after registration is when you quickly develop your skills in the workplace and become part of the team. Year 2 is usually when midwives start thinking about progression and how to map out their future career.

Progression can take you into many different areas of midwifery employment and you need to start with yourself and consider where your strengths and interests lie. Are there particular areas of your work that you really enjoy and others that you would rather not do too often? Are there clinical areas where you would like to build up your expertise? Would you like to learn new skills that could take you into new environments such as management? Keep an account of your thoughts and discuss them with your line manager at your personal development review as they may have further ideas and suggestions to make.

Midwifery posts beyond Level 6 can take you in many directions. As well as being an excellent practitioner you will be expected to focus and develop further skills at an advanced level. You may enjoy organising, planning and developing systems and staff. If this is you, you might consider a managerial post such as a midwifery team leader in a labour or postnatal ward. Such a post would include being responsible for the day-to-day management of the midwifery services in your ward. You would lead the team, organise workloads and ensure that care is effectively delivered with the resources available. Staff recruitment and development would also be part of your remit. You would continue to practise as a midwife and act as a professional lead in your ward, providing advice to other midwives and health professionals when required. This type of higher-level post is great if you enjoy being busy and focused, dealing with competing demands for your support and ideas on a continuous basis. It may be the type of post that would suit you if you enjoy developing processes and ensuring that services are delivered to a high standard.

> According to the Office for National Statistics, in 2008 there were 19,639 full-time equivalent midwives in England alone.

You may have enjoyed teaching and supporting women and their families in your career to date. You may also like to focus on a particular aspect of midwifery and develop your expertise in a specific clinical area. Advanced practitioner posts such as lead midwife for breastfeeding would be worth considering if this is the direction in which you would like to steer your career. As a lead midwife you would be expected to promote breastfeeding within the maternity unit to midwives, allied health professionals and the wider community. You would have developmental responsibilities and be expected to devise and lead on new ways of working. You would also be expected to collect, analyse and disseminate data to show how your area of responsibility is developing. There would be a training element to your work: you would be teaching staff working with mothers. Alongside these duties, you would continue to practise as a midwife and act as a role model for new and experienced staff. Advanced practitioner posts such as this are suitable for anyone who is a good clinician and a confident communicator who enjoys working with a wide variety of people, from women and their families to professionals in health care and related services. It is the type of role that needs someone who also has strong organisational and project development skills.

Returning to higher education as a lecturer is another role that experienced midwives move into. If you enjoy learning you can continue to enhance your education by studying for a master's degree and then for a PhD. If you enjoy research and teaching, career opportunities exist as lecturers and subsequently professors of midwifery in universities. Such careers would immerse you in the clinical development and education of new midwives. This would involve one-to-one support, running tutorials and lectures. You would also be expected to conduct research on areas of midwifery in which you had a professional interest.

Midwifery roles

Looking at the variety of job titles in midwifery provides a glimpse of the variety of career possibilities for those with a few years of clinical experience:

- birth centre team leader

- infant feeding co-ordinator

- in-patient midwife co-ordinator

- Sure Start midwife

- delivery suite manager

- consultant midwife

- advanced midwifery practitioner for mental health and learning needs.

Birgit Gray, Senior Community Midwife, Hampshire: Level 7

I trained as a nurse and then a midwife at the Royal County Hospital in Winchester. While on my nursing training I realised that I really enjoyed my obstetrics placements and that I was looking for a career where I could be my own practitioner, working under a professional code of practice but also able to make decisions. I therefore decided to train as a midwife as I enjoyed working with women and being a part of a special time in their lives.

My first post was as a hospital midwife, working on postnatal, antenatal and labour wards. Having gained experience I became a senior midwife and labour ward sister for 16 years. As a co-ordinator and manager, I missed delivering babies and working more directly with women so I undertook two maternity covers in the community and moved over to being a community midwife in 1998.

As a senior community midwife I have a caseload of 60 women a year and carry out all their antenatal care, plus running one clinic a week. I also carry out postnatal care and am on call for home births, of which I may be involved in six to 10 a year. My other duties include attending meetings with colleagues and other health and social care professionals, including doctors, social workers, health visitors and perinatal mental health staff. As a senior midwife I carry out annual staff appraisals and mentor students.

The benefit of being a community midwife is that you are able to plan your own day and get to know the women you work with and their families throughout their pregnancy. You are part of a team providing good care to women and getting to know

them as they progress in their pregnancy and being aware
of any complications that may arise. During home births, for
example, you need to know what is normal for a mother and
when they need to be referred.

In order to be effective in this role you have to be flexible,
adaptable and able to adjust to situations quickly. You need to
be a good communicator and an advocate for the mother who
will represent her requests to other professionals. You have
to be open minded and build up trust with a wide variety of
people from differing backgrounds.

The role can be challenging and you have to be accountable
to yourself and your code of practice. You need to be able to
be on call and have the energy to work through home births,
which are intense.

FURTHER PROFESSIONAL EDUCATION

Whichever way your career develops you may find that you want to
continue studying, either immediately after completing your degree or
diploma or a few years later. The NHS Careers Framework encourages
nurses and midwives to develop their skills through training courses and
other learning opportunities. Nursing and midwifery posts at Level 7 and
beyond are also increasingly asking for higher-level qualifications, such
as master's degrees. Outside the NHS employers also want their staff to
be well trained, which is especially important if they need to maintain their
NMC registration. For many nurses and midwives it is simply the case
that they enjoy learning and will look to further and higher education for
further development.

Further education colleges run short part-time courses in a wide range
of subject areas. Topics on offer are wide ranging and cover short clinical
courses on subjects such as dementia care through to specialist interests

such as massage and counselling skills. Visit local college websites for information on the range of part-time courses on offer in your area.

A wide range of higher-level postgraduate courses are available at universities for qualified nurses and midwives who wish to enhance their skills or training. Anyone who has completed a diploma course in nursing can top up their qualification to a degree through part-time study while in nursing employment. This can be done within five years of qualifying and needs to be agreed with their line manager. For those wanting to expand their professional knowledge, master's degree courses and postgraduate diplomas are available in subjects such as:

■ public health practice

■ mental health studies

■ advanced nursing practice

■ leadership and management in health care.

Some nurses and midwives decide that they want to research in far greater depth a specific area of clinical interest and subsequently opt to read for a PhD.

Career progression for nurses and midwives can be dynamic and varied. This chapter has attempted to give a flavour of the options available after having worked in a Level 5 post for a number of years. The challenges faced by health care providers, such as the NHS, as well as its general staffing and salary structure, have been touched on. The range of more senior nursing and midwifery jobs, along with the responsibilities associated with these posts, has been included to provide an insight into future options available to those entering either profession.

Chapter Twelve
FURTHER INFORMATION

This book has provided an insight into employment and training in nursing and midwifery and many organisations and professional bodies have been mentioned that support these topics.

NURSING AND MIDWIFERY PROFESSIONAL REPRESENTATIVES

Nursing and Midwifery Council
23 Portland Place, London W1B 1PZ
Tel: 020 7333 9333 (registration and professional advice)
www.nmc-uk.org

Royal College of Nursing
20 Cavendish Square, London W1G 0RN
Tel: 020 7409 3333
www.rcn.org.uk

Royal College of Midwives
15 Mansfield Street, London W1G 9NH
Tel: 020 7312 3535
www.rcm.org.uk

An Bord Altranais (Irish nursing board)
18/20 Carysfort Avenue, Blackrock, Co. Dublin, Ireland
Tel: 00353 1639 8500
www.nursingboard.ie

PROFESSIONAL PUBLICATIONS

Nursing Times
Weekly magazine for nurses in the UK.
www.nursingtimes.net

Midwives
Bi-monthly midwifery magazine of the Royal College of Midwives.
www.rcm.org.uk/midwives

Nursing Standard
The magazine of the Royal College of Nursing.
http://nursingstandard.rcnpublishing.co.uk

PROFESSIONAL TRAINING

Universities and Colleges Admissions Service (UCAS)
Rosehill, New Barn Lane, Cheltenham, Gloucestershire GL52 3LZ
Tel: 0871 468 0 468 (customer service unit)
www.ucas.com

CAREERS ADVICE

NHS Careers
Tel: 0345 606 0655 (helpline)
www.nhscareers.nhs.uk

What Can I Do With My Degree?
NHS Careers-aided guidance site providing career ideas for graduates
wishing to work in the NHS.
www.whatcanidowithmydegree.nhs.uk

Prospects

Careers information and advice website for undergraduates and graduates. Full of useful information on all careers and a great section on careers in the health care sector.
www.prospects.ac.uk

Forces careers websites

Army: www.armyjobs.mod.uk
Royal Navy: www.royalnavy.mod.uk/careers
Royal Air Force: www.raf.mod.uk/careers

Chapter Thirteen
GLOSSARY

Acute care: short-term hospital treatment for a severe episode of illness, disease or injury. It can refer to any area of nursing practice, including adult (e.g. people with pneumonia – acute medical care; appendicitis – acute surgical care); children's (e.g. a child dehydrated from diarrhoea; a child with a burn injury); mental health (e.g. a person with psychosis or paranoia). Acute care can also be called urgent and unscheduled care.

Ambulatory: refers to 'walking about' – typically patients who can walk themselves to a clinic or around a hospital.

Anaesthetic: a drug that causes lack of feeling or awareness by interfering with nerves (e.g. a local anaesthetic affects one part of the body, such as a hand or leg). The widely known 'general anaesthetic' artificially induces a controlled loss of consciousness (being 'put to sleep'), most commonly so that a person is pain free and not aware of a surgical procedure.

Anatomy: the study of the structures of the body, from cellular to skeletal.

Antenatal: the care of pregnant women prior to the birth of the baby – in other words, up to the time of labour and delivery.

Appendicitis: the appendix is a tiny structure near the start of the large intestine which contributes to immunity and maintaining normal bacteria in the bowel. Appendicitis occurs when the appendix becomes blocked and infected, causing severe pain, acute illness and often a range of typical signs. If it is untreated, rapid deterioration occurs, but early routine surgery is highly successful with no long-term effects.

Auscultation: listening to internal sounds in the body, normally using a manual or electronic stethoscope. It can be used to help examine the heart for the opening and closing of the heart valves and flow; the lungs and airways to hear where and how air is moving and which parts of the lungs are expanding; the gastrointestinal system (all of the bowel) to assess movement and function. Auscultation needs a lot of practice before you become confident in its use. A very interesting website is www.auscultation.com, which has accompanying sounds!

Bilirubin: is a bile pigment that is a by-product of the breakdown of haemoglobin in the liver. Too much bilirubin causes the skin to yellow.

Bipolar disorder: affects how a person feels physically and mentally, with altered thoughts, feelings, perceptions and behaviour. Many – but not all – patients also experience extreme swings in mood from 'high' (mania) to 'low' (depression), with varying degrees of severity – this part of the illness used to be called manic depression. It is a long-term mental health condition.

Blood transfusion: essentially transfers blood from one person to another, but it involves complex laboratory checking of compatibility first. Occasionally whole blood is transfused, but more frequently the components of donated blood are separated, each part – for example red cells, plasma or platelets – being used separately. Blood transfusions are used for some routine surgery, after severe trauma and blood loss and regularly for some people with anaemia or haemophilia. Blood transfusions are delivered intravenously.

Cannulation: a cannula is a fine plastic tube. Of the many diverse types and uses, by far the most common is a venous cannula inserted into a vein to deliver fluid or drugs or to take blood samples. Cannulation (putting the cannula in) is a skill frequently used by midwives and also by nurses in many settings. Although widely used, care must be taken to avoid infection and other complications.

Cardiovascular: illnesses or treatments described as affecting the cardiovascular system are referring to issues affecting any part of the blood circulation system – from the pump (heart) to the major delivery blood vessels (arteries), peripheral blood vessels in the skin, tissues and organs (capillaries) and 'return' blood vessels (veins). It also refers to the control mechanisms of the system, including the electrical conduction system of the heart. Cardiovascular illnesses include hypertension (high blood pressure); hypotension (low blood pressure); angina (pain caused by lack of oxygen in the arteries supplying the cardiac muscle) and myocardial infarction (death of cardiac muscle – sometimes called a heart attack).

CCU (coronary care unit): a specialist unit supporting people who, for example, have had a heart attack, have angina that is difficult to control with medication, have heart failure (the heart is not pumping enough blood) or who have a disordered electrical conduction system in their heart.

Cognitive behavioural therapy: is a therapy aimed at helping the patient understand what is happening in their life and what they would like to be different.

Community matron: usually nurses, from any branch, who case manage patients with complex needs and long-term conditions in their own homes. The aim is to prevent unnecessary and expensive hospital admissions and facilitate early discharge from hospital. Community matrons are experienced nurses who have gained additional qualifications in patient assessment, decision making, clinical leadership and prescribing; they are among the most senior nurses working regularly with patients in the UK.

COPD (chronic obstructive pulmonary disease): describes a number of conditions including chronic bronchitis (inflamed/infected airways in the lungs) and emphysema (collapsed or destroyed air sacs in the lungs). In COPD the airways in the lungs become narrower, making it more difficult to breathe air in or expel breath out. COPD is a long-term condition, one of the most common in the UK. It cannot be reversed but is often controlled with medication, physiotherapy and other support. Some people with COPD also have asthma (narrowing of the airways caused by local muscle contraction), which, while dangerous, can often be controlled with drugs. The word 'chronic' means that the problem is long term.

Critical care: the care of people with acute, life-threatening disorders, both planned and emergency. Critical care takes place in intensive care units, trauma/accident centres, anaesthetic and recovery rooms, coronary care units, maternity delivery rooms, etc. Nurses working in critical care units often have to respond to situations very quickly; care may variously involve support for breathing (ventilator); renal/kidney function (dialysis); a failing heart (mechanical assistance). Critical care units usually have a nurse–patient ratio of one to one.

Domiciliary care: care delivered in the person's normal 'domicile' or place of residence; most community care can be described as domiciliary.

ECG (electrocardiogram): records tiny changes in electrical activity in the muscle of the heart (the myocardium) – this can be done continuously to be read as a 'trace' on a monitor (particularly useful for detecting changes in the rhythm of the heart) or in more detail as a single assessment (particularly to evaluate damage to the myocardium). An ECG machine only 'reads' the electrical activity of the heart – it doesn't change it in any way.

HDU (high dependency unit): these can be found in hospitals supporting adults or children with either physical or mental ill health. HDUs are often described as a 'step-up' or 'step-down' unit – between a general ward and an intensive or critical care unit. People in an HDU generally need frequent assessment and more concentrated care than is typical of a general ward, but without the life support equipment of intensive care. HDUs have a high staff–patient ratio.

Holistic care: universally promoted in nursing and midwifery, holistic care recognises that all aspects of a person should be considered in order to care for the person as a whole. This means carefully taking into account not just their immediate physical or mental health needs but also all psychological, physical, social and spiritual needs. Also considered is the idea of maximising independence for the individual.

Injections: used to give small volumes of fluid to a patient, almost always solutions of drugs. There are many types of injection – intravenous (into a vein); intramuscular (into muscle); subcutaneous (just under the skin); intradermal (into the skin), etc. Many types of drug can be given: some are regularly self-administered by patients themselves (e.g. insulin for people who have diabetes); others by nurses and midwives (e.g. strong antibiotics or analgesics, or in emergency situations).

Interprofessional practice: has long been talked about in professional health care but it is only since 2004 that it has become a significant component of many health courses leading to professional registration. It refers to two or more professions working together with a common purpose, collaboration and commitment. This book has referred to a very broad range of health professionals whom nurses and midwives work with to support people in need – this is not only now fully established in 'real practice' but also something which will expand further in coming years. Linked terms, often used interchangeably, include 'interdisciplinary', 'multidisciplinary' and 'transdisciplinary'.

Intrapartum: the period of childbirth or delivery.

Intravenous fluids/infusion: given to maintain or restore correct body fluid levels when people are unable to do so themselves. Typically this might be in children who are dehydrated; in infection; during surgery; for people who are unconscious; for people unable to swallow or absorb fluid normally. Often called a drip. Fluids are given through a cannula inserted into a vein; a pump is normally used to regulate the flow. The type of fluid given can be adjusted according to the patient's needs.

Intubation: placing an artificial tube into the body. In practice almost always refers to tracheal intubation – placing a flexible plastic tube into the trachea to either protect the airway (e.g. if the patient is unconscious) or as a way of artificially ventilating (inflating) the lungs (e.g. during an anaesthetic or after severe trauma). Can be used in people of all ages/ sizes.

Life support equipment: equipment needed to sustain life when people are critically ill or injured (their life is at risk). Typically such equipment is used in trauma units and intensive care units and may include a ventilator (to artificially inflate the lungs); intravenous infusions; complex monitoring equipment to continually assess the heart, brain, venous return and arterial blood pressure/oxygen saturation; kidney dialysis; heart/lung bypass (artificial heart); complex drug treatments.

Mentoring: two (or more) people working together to further learning and development of skills and to challenge and extend personal development. Mentoring is a key part of nursing and midwifery courses where on each placement the student is closely linked with a mentor (trained and experienced) and often with a second registered health professional, who acts as a 'buddy mentor'.

Metabolic or metabolism: refers to biochemical processes. These are complex, involving multiple interactions, and include anabolism (the building up or creation of substances such as noradrenaline, which is involved in transmitting nerve impulses and controlling blood pressure) and catabolism (the breakdown of substances, e.g. glucose is broken down to release energy in the body). Metabolic disorders include diabetes (insufficient insulin, needed to regulate the glucose in our cells) and acromegaly (excess growth hormone).

Neonatal: the first four weeks after birth.

Neurological: illnesses or treatments: refers to issues connected to the nervous system, either the central nervous system (brain and spinal cord) or the peripheral nervous system (the distributed nerves to skin, limbs and organs).

Nutritional supplements: additions to or replacement of the normal diet, often to provide vital nutrients that a person cannot eat or cannot absorb adequately. They may take the form of high-protein drinks or foods; complete nutrition delivered directly into the stomach or bowel by an artificial tube via nose or abdomen (enteral nutrition); full intravenous nutrition delivered by a drip and pump directly into the person's veins (parenteral nutrition).

Oxygen saturation: the measure of how much oxygen the blood is carrying in the arteries; 100% being the maximum the haemoglobin in red blood cells can carry. On a results sheet the term SaO2 is normally used; the abbreviation 'sates' is not an approved one. Oxygen saturation below 90% is normally unhealthy and may cause cyanosis (blue/grey-tinged lips and extremities); this needs prompt attention.

Palliative care: any health care intended to reduce the severity of symptoms (for example pain) rather than providing a cure or slowing progression of a disease. Palliative care aims to minimise suffering and improve quality of life rather than routinely planning to extend life as long as possible.

Perfusionist: is a member of the open heart surgery team, responsible for the heart–lung machine, who ensures the patient receives enough oxygen through their blood.

Perinatal: the time immediately before and/or after birth.

Pharmacist: a qualified and registered professional practitioner able to formulate and dispense drugs/medications; provide clinical information on drugs or medications to health professionals and patients; and (in the UK and elsewhere) offer a range of health advice, including advice on sexual health and smoking cessation.

Pharmacology: the study of drugs, how they are made, their effects on the body and their administration.

Physiology: the study of how the body functions, for example processes such as digestion, blood flow and pain. It is important for nurses and midwives to have a good understanding of physiology – it is taught on all courses – as it closely links to clinical decisions concerned with blood pressure, wound healing, pain management, etc.

Postnatal: the period immediately after birth of the baby until the child is about one month old. During this period a mother's altered 'pregnancy physiology' returns to pre-pregnancy status. In the postnatal period the baby begins to learn and to interact with the environment; a key midwifery role is to assess the health of mother and baby and the parenting involved, including baby nutrition/breastfeeding.

Pre-eclampsia: occurs in pregnant women who have both hypertension and the presence of protein in their urine (a sign of developing kidney damage). Pre-eclampsia can be mild, in which case the woman's health is carefully monitored and rest advised; or severe, which may result in damage to her kidneys and/or liver. Where the health of either mother or baby is thought to be at risk delivery is often induced or a caesarian section (operation to deliver the baby surgically) is performed.

Psoriasis: a skin condition in which the cells replace themselves too quickly. There are many types of psoriasis but a typical form is patches of red and crusty skin around joints or in the scalp, which are often uncomfortable and itchy. Psoriasis is a long-term condition with periodic exacerbations, helped by a variety of medications.

Resuscitation: an emergency procedure for people whose heart has stopped (cardiac arrest – mostly adults) or who have stopped breathing (respiratory arrest – adults or children), or both. CPR is the abbreviation for cardio-pulmonary resuscitation – the process of compressing the chest and artificially ventilating (inflating) the lungs. Resuscitation can be learned by almost anyone and is a really useful skill to have for the public as well as health professionals; it is always taught to a high standard on all nursing and midwifery courses.

Schizophrenia: a severe mental disorder in which people experience agitation, delusions and (non-drug-induced) hallucinations, all of which contribute to disordered patterns of thought. Schizophrenia affects about 1% of the population. Treatment involves medication and nurse-led therapies.

Venesection: entering a vein with a cannula or needle to withdraw blood. More formally, it refers to removing quite a lot of blood – perhaps 500ml or more – for people who have too much iron or too many cells in their blood. In common practice, however, it also refers to taking small amounts of blood for testing – typically 10 to 30ml in an adult. Venesection is sometimes undertaken by trained technicians but often by nurses and midwives.

Venous return: the flow of blood from all over the body back to the heart, from where it is pumped to the lungs to be re-oxygenated. Blood in the venous system (veins) has low oxygen saturation as the oxygen has been used, for example in our muscles, and is darker coloured than the bright red blood of arteries. Blood in the veins is under low pressure, unlike blood in the arteries, which is under high pressure.

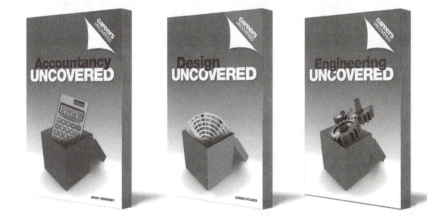
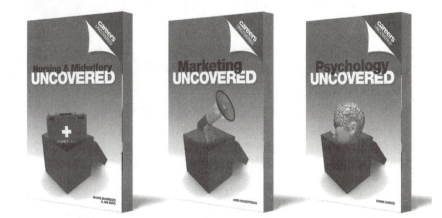
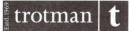

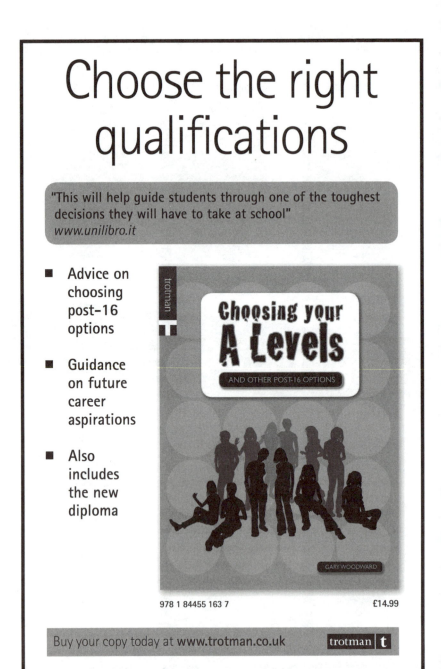

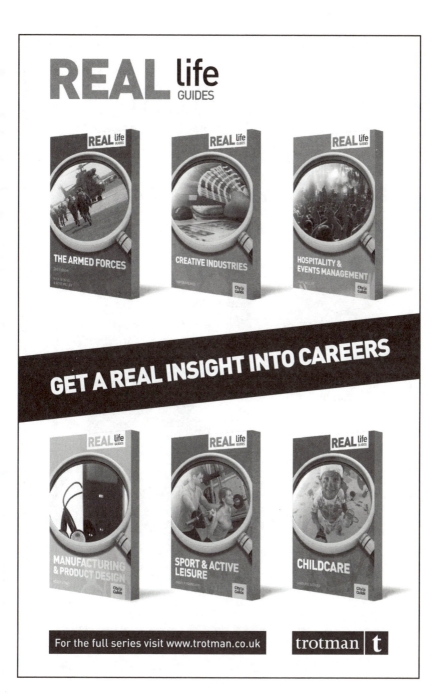

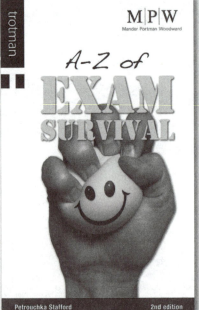